Disease and Medicine in W̶ History

Disease and Medicine in World History is a concise introduction to diverse ideas about diseases and their treatment throughout the world. Drawing on case studies from ancient Egypt to present-day America, Asia and Europe, this survey discusses concepts of sickness and forms of treatment in many cultures. Sheldon Watts shows that many medical systems in the past were shaped as much by philosophers and metaphysicians as by university-trained doctors and other practitioners.

This volume is a landmark contribution to the field of world history. It covers the principal medical systems known in the past, based on extensive original research. Watts raises questions about globalization in medicine and the potential impact of infectious diseases in the present day.

Subjects covered include:

- pharaonic Egypt and the pre-conquest New World;
- the evolution of medical systems in the Middle East;
- health and healing on the Indian subcontinent;
- medicine and disease in China;
- the globalization of disease in the modern world;
- the birth and evolution of modern scientific medicine.

Sheldon Watts is the author of *Epidemics and History: Disease, Power and Imperialism* (Yale, 1997). He has served as Senior Lecturer in History at the University of Ilorin, Nigeria and visiting Associate Professor of History at the American University in Cairo.

Themes in World History
Series editor: Peter N. Stearns

The *Themes in World History* series offers focused treatment of a range of human experiences and institutions in the world history context. The purpose is to provide serious, if brief, discussions of important topics as additions to textbook coverage and document collections. The treatments will allow students to probe particular facets of the human story in greater depth than textbook coverage allows, and to gain a fuller sense of historians' analytical methods and debates in the process. Each topic is handled over time – allowing discussions of changes and continuities. Each topic is assessed in terms of a range of different societies and religions – allowing comparisons of relevant similarities and differences. Each book in the series helps readers deal with world history in action, evaluating global contexts as they work through some of the key components of human society and human life.

Gender in World History
Peter N. Stearns

Consumerism in World History
Peter N. Stearns

Warfare in World History
Michael S. Neiberg

Disease and Medicine in World History
Sheldon Watts

Asian Democracy in World History
Alan T. Wood

Disease and Medicine in World History

Sheldon Watts

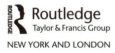

Routledge
Taylor & Francis Group

NEW YORK AND LONDON

First published 2003
by Routledge
29 West 35th Street, New York, NY 10001

Simultaneously published in the UK
by Routledge
11 New Fetter Lane, London EC4P 4EE

Routledge is an imprint of the Taylor & Francis Group

Typeset in Garamond by
Florence Production Ltd, Stoodleigh, Devon
Printed and bound in Great Britain by
MPG Books Ltd, Bodmin, Cornwall

Library of Congress Cataloging in Publication Data
Watts, S. J. (Sheldon J.)
  Disease and medicine in world history / Sheldon Watts.
    p. cm.
  Includes bibliographical references and index.
  1. Medicine–History. I. Title.
  R131 .W35 2003
  610′.9—dc21   2002153796

British Library Cataloguing in Publication Data
A catalogue record for this book is available from the British Library

ISBN 0–415–27816–3 (hbk)
ISBN 0–415–27817–1 (pbk)

To my students in the West, in Nigeria and in Egypt

Contents

Preface

In the last 15 years or so, the discipline of World History has finally come of age. Before that time, courses listed in college catalogs as "world history" tended to be little more than the history of western Europe and America. Though short sections did of course deal with Non-western history, their main apparent purpose was to explain the mess the rest of the world had been in before it was "rescued" by the progressive West.

Nowadays, this Eurocentric perspective has been tossed over the side. It has been replaced by a Global History which at least aims to be more truly universal. Among its other attributes, this new global history recognizes that the real world in times past consisted of a very large number of culture groups, each of which was distinct and separate from the others.

Within this short book, limitations of space permit me only to touch on certain medical aspects of five or six Non-western societies or sets of societies: ancient Egypt and native pre-Columbian America, the Islamic Middle East, India, China. Ancient Greece – when seen from *some* (not all) disciplinary perspectives – was also a Non-western society. As will be demonstrated, each of these societies (or groupings of societies) developed a cluster of formal medical systems which co-existed with various forms of empirical medicine.

Given that World History is essentially a new discipline, so too is *Medical History* as the field is now coming to be understood. In the old days most medical history was written in the West by retired medical doctors or by nationalist historians whose primary aim was to glorify the great medical men of the past. The names of these heroes were engraved on the cornices of monumental buildings like the London School of Tropical Medicine and Hygiene – where they can still be seen today.

However, my own conceptualization of the subject has little to do with "great men." As a medico-cultural historian, I regard all past approaches to sickness and healing as aspects of the great diversity which always has been a core aspect of *Homo sapiens sapiens* (humankind).

Acknowledgments

This book incorporates my own interpretations of the findings of scores of medical and cultural historians: to all of them I am most grateful.

My especial thanks to the World Historians and Medical Historians who have given me encouragement in this and in similar projects over the years. These scholars include: Peter N. Stearns of George Mason University, academic editor of the Themes in World History Series; Jerry H. Bentley of The University of Hawai'i, editor of the *Journal of World History*; Gert H. Brieger of The Johns Hopkins Institute for the History of Medicine, editor of the *Bulletin of the History of Medicine*, and Roy Porter, until his recent untimely death, the leading historian of medicine at the Wellcome Institute for the History of Medicine, in London.

The Egyptologists, Dimitri Meeks and Christine Favard-Meeks, made helpful comments on a longer draft of parts of Chapter 2, Ancient Egypt. Professor Ruth Mayer, Dr Brigitte Weingart and other participants at the Virus! Conference held in Bonn, Germany 17–19 January 2002, offered insightful comments on aspects of Chapter 7, "The globalization of disease after 1450." To all of these scholars I am most grateful.

My wife, Susan Watts, a medical geographer, has read and critically commented upon each draft chapter as it emerged from the computer. She has always been most generous with her time, and with Conradian and all other forms of support. Without her this project would never have been brought to completion.

Cairo
October 2002

Chapter I

Sickness and health, a global concern

The big picture

This book is based on the understanding that during the last 5,000 years, each cultural grouping on planet earth has had its own clustering of ways in which to explain and to treat what they perceived as various categories of disease and illness. Disease history thus alerts us to the diversity of the human experience.

Another, quite different, reason for study of the history of disease and medicine is to pick up background information on why there is such a huge disparity in the health status of different human groupings in the world today. As the World Health Organization and other authorities assure us, at the present time the standard of living and health status of one fifth of humanity is no better than it was 2,000 years ago during the long era when Roman Imperial agents held most of the Western world in thrall. As mention of these disparities reminds us, throughout history the exercise of power over the many by the few (through the use of soldiers, the use of distributors of doctrine and information, and the use of tax collectors) has commonly been found in socially-stratified societies. It was not, however, much found among groupings consisting solely of hunter-gatherers and nomads.

In addition to the continuities just mentioned, there have also been many important discontinuities in the history of civilized societies. The discontinuity of most immediate concern to us here was the invention of modern biomedicine itself. To some people it may come as a surprise to learn that modern scientific medicine is a recent invention of the West which only dates from the late 1860s, 1870s and 1880s. Little more than a century and a quarter old, it owes its existence to the seminal work of half a dozen men, among them Louis Pasteur of France (with his work on rabies and fermentation), and Robert Koch of north Germany, discoverer of the tiny, living causal agent of cholera – the cholera vibrio. Koch also discovered the causal agent of tuberculosis, the causal agent of anthrax and several other diseases.

As I will demonstrate more fully in Chapter 9, what really differentiates modern scientific medicine from all other medical systems is that it works within a conceptual framework which owed remarkably little to anything that had existed before either in Western Europe or in Europe's intellectual seed-bed, the Middle East. Biomedicine (struggling to be born in the 1860s) owed even less to the medical systems existing at that time in China and in India. (On India and China see Chapters 5 and 6.)

One idea central to the new conceptual web which was biomedicine, was disease specificity. This held, among other things, that infant diarrhea, for example, was a set of symptoms caused by specific pathogens which could not transform themselves into the causal agent of another distinct disease such as cholera – even though both were symptomatized by runny bowels. Another idea central to the new conceptual web was that a *specific* disease causal agent (for example, the microscopic living causal agent of malaria or of cholera or another infectious disease) was the necessary and sufficient cause of the disease when it struck a particular victim/sufferer. No other causes (for example, the pre-existing mental state of the victim, or his/her economic status) were, strictly speaking, of any interest to modern scientific medicine.

Having said this we must be aware that people in the present-day West (which in terms of science includes Japan) live in the post-modern era and that some of the "modern" ideas that were created in order to come to terms with infectious diseases caused by bacterial agents which could be seen under a microscope are now on the edge of being superceded. At present, new paradigms concern themselves with things like viruses (which are host-dependent rather than independent beings like bacteria), and with chronic disease conditions brought on by what was once thought to be old age, but which now are seen as genetically related (see Chapter 10). Yet, as of the year 2003, the old infectious diseases (sometimes in the form of new mutants) are still the leading cause of death among humanity at large. This means that many of the lessons of nineteenth-century medicine about disease control, and about the essential nature of a pure water supply and sanitation, are still highly relevant.

Another thing distinctive about modern scientific medicine (in practical terms, newly invented in the years after 1865) was that its key insights were derived from work done in the *laboratory*. Within the laboratory, medical scientists used what were, in effect, new tools (among them, an improved microscope which was soon superceded by a more sophisticated instrument, which was, in turn, superceded by one even more sophisticated), and new techniques (staining, for instance) in order to test in detail particular facets of their new range of hypotheses about the causal agents of disease and how these agents behaved when they came into contact with humankind.

Our new understanding of the shortness of the period of time which encompasses the actual past of applied science in general (beginning a little more than 200 years ago with the use of the new science of chemistry to create new dyes for cloth) and of biomedicine (with a past of less than 150 years) has all but replaced the old orthodoxy. The old notion held that in the West, modern science and medicine both had deep roots that went back in an undeviating and continuous straight line to the very beginnings of western civilization. Fortunately, (for the credibility of the historical profession) in recent years this mythic past has now been shown for what it is. It has been replaced by increasing awareness of the discontinuities which marked the human experience in the western EurAsian lands in the last 3,000 years.

Looking at matters from a broad perspective, the standard position of twenty-first century World Historians is to remind readers that the *content* of what is considered to be "science" and what is considered to be "medicine" varies very much, both in time and in place, from one setting to another. Going beyond content, they also realize that the words themselves have undergone shifts in meaning.

For example, the English-language word "science" and the French-language "science" are both derived from the Latin word for "knowledge," *scientia*. During most of its history of usage in the West, the word "science" could mean metaphysical "knowledge," or a philosopher's "knowledge," or practical "knowledge" or a mixture of all three. In Britain, well into the 1870s and 1880s, learned writers continued to be rather vague about what they meant when using the word. By "science" some meant knowledge of the sort authenticated by Ancient writers, while others meant knowledge in the sense of the new, functionally useful and plausible scientific hypotheses derived from the laboratory, repeated testing and so on, which is to say, "modern science" and modern "scientific medicine." But out in the far reaches of Empire, vagueness about what was meant by "scientific medicine" continued to serve the purposes of tax-collecting colonial authority well into the 1920s.

Yet, though modern scientific medicine (biomedicine) is an invention of the West, it must also be acknowledged that in the Non-west, and globally, before the 1860s there were a host of other ways of attempting to meet the challenges posed by disease, and indeed of defining what was meant by disease. The road to understanding the totality of the human experience (world history) lies through accepting the need for a pluralistic approach.

This is another way of saying that the Chinese and the Indian and the African and Pacific Islands' medical systems in existence around 1650 – before these societies were placed under threat by aggressive traders and military personnel from western Europe and North America – can only be understood in terms of their own cultures. They cannot properly be interpreted as being merely erroneous gropings after the (mythic) universal, ultimate medical truth, which happened to come into the possession of western Europe and North America during the years when Western Imperialism and rampant militarism were at their triumphalist height, 1860–1914. Instead, each of these medical systems (or more accurately, groupings of systems) – Indian, Chinese, Middle Eastern, Native American – must be seen as having had its own logic and its own integrity. Each demonstrated the diversity of human inventiveness and human aspiration and thus is of equal interest to the world historian.

Humans as cultural beings and as biological beings: a disputed frontier

As medical anthropologists remind us, humankind has two attributes that are closely interlinked, yet separate. Humans are biological entities (we are an animal type known among ourselves as *Homo sapiens sapiens*), while at the same time we are the bearers of culture. Turning briefly to the first attribute: as biological entities, we are all ultimately descended from human ancestors who lived in Africa. As is well known, some of our ancestors remained on that continent, others migrated to Asia, Australia and Europe. Going on from Asia, some of our ancestors eventually migrated to the Americas. Much later, some of the European ancestors migrated to the New World where, in time, they were joined by more recent immigrants from Asia.

But when seen from the point of view of germs, microbes, viruses and other living disease causal agents, as well as from the point of view of non-living agencies of death (such as meteorites), all human beings are pretty much alike, by virtue of their basic biology. In the right circumstances, all human beings, universally, across the globe, could be adversely affected by killing causal agent "x" or "y." To illustrate this point, rather than saying anything more here about the influenza epidemic of 1918–19 which killed off great numbers of people everywhere in the world (perhaps 21 million all told), let us turn to a non-living agency of death which did its work long before proto humans had evolved in Africa.

It is now known that a destructive causal agent appeared in the Western hemisphere 65 million years ago in the form of a large meteorite which crashed down into the Yucatan peninsula, blocking out the sun. Deprived of life-giving light for several months (or years) all but the smallest living things became extinct. Here, then, was a case of their basic biology (reptiles' dependence on organic materials for food) working *against* survival.

Yet, in more recent times, mammals' biology works *for* species survival. More specifically, within the human body there are a wide variety of protective devices – including an immune system containing antibodies against specific kinds of infection – which the brain, once triggered, sets in motion against an invading alien force. Within the human body there are also biological forces – related to the immune system – working to heal injured body parts. Long before modern medical scientists began to study these processes, curers and medical persons recognized (though not always explicitly) that nature itself was the most reliable of all healing agents. Before the advent of antibiotics in 1943 (and sometimes even now) the most that health counselors, medical doctors and attendant family members could hope for was that they would be able to keep the sick person alive long enough for nature to effect a cure.

In the chapters that follow, the role of nature – the in-built curative powers of the human body itself – should always be kept in mind. As a corollary of this, it should be recognized that if the various human cultural groupings we will examine had been dependent solely on the curative powers of their own medicines and treatments when confronted with disease, humankind would long since have become extinct. As it is, nature prevailed often enough over interfering humans to ensure group survival. Once sick people recovered – very often *despite* the medicines and treatments inflicted on them by healers – some of the youthful ones went on to contribute to the gene bank of their ethnic or tribal group.

Mention of genes brings us to another aspect of the biological identity of humankind – the possibility of genetic modification, a process not yet entirely understood. Exemplifying one approach, it is now held that human groupings that have been exposed over the centuries to unfavorable environmental conditions in a semi-arid setting who confront long periods without much in the way of food develop an ability to survive; this ability is perhaps inherited.

A good example are the still surviving (but much threatened) aboriginals of Australia (all 200,000 of them, the remnants of people who settled that island continent 60,000 or so years ago). In the short term, during times of stress, Australian aboriginals seem to have adopted the technique of cutting down on all unnecessary exercise during daylight hours. But in the long term, over 60 millennia, possibly through the processes of adaptive evolution, these people's genes (or so it seems) toned their bodily functions in such a way that they could survive longish periods of hardship with little food. In our own time (early twenty-first century), when people of this sort are brought into Sydney, Melbourne and other modern Australian cities and fed junk food, their health rapidly deteriorates. According to the biological interpretation, this is because their genes don't equip them with the ability to cope with the new diet.

However – given that the Human Genome project is still in its early days – this information from Australia has yet to be collated with information from deprived areas in the West (such as working-class neighborhoods in Glasgow) where young people apparently bearing only Celtic, Norse and Anglo-Saxon genes also seem unable to cope with junk food: living on nothing else they become sluggish and obese. In this instance culture (working-class habits) seems to have the upper hand over genetic inheritance. These somewhat contradictory findings can only lead us to conclude that the terrain between the two interpretations (humans as biological beings and humans as bearers of culture) is still very much in dispute.

This also alerts us to the possibility that so-called biological facts (which on closer inspection are often little more than prejudice) have sometimes altered outsiders' perceptions of who was, or was not, prone to a particular disease. These erroneous perceptions have sometimes led to huge social consequences. This was unfortunately true in the case of West Africans and of their captors, the white-skinned profiteers who invaded their lands and established the transatlantic slave trade early in the sixteenth century. Following onwards from the long era of Black-African slavery in the New World, several old-style historians of medicine held that sub-Saharan Africa was the place of origin of many of the most lethal of the diseases that came to plague the West, and that these diseases had been brought to the West in the bodies of enslaved persons. They did not consider the possibility that these diseases might have been brought in in the bodies of white-skinned slave-ship crew who were in the employ of European-based entrepreneurs.

Disease evolution

In recent years, one of the most disturbing findings of medical scientists, paleontologists and evolutionary biologists is that disease types are not constant over time. Of especial concern to us here are hypotheses about the comparatively recent evolution of many of the infectious diseases that now threaten humankind. The human immunodeficiency virus (HIV), discovered in 1981, is simply one of the last of these mutations to have been identified (Chapter 10).

One suggested cause of disease evolution during late pre-historic (pre-literate) and early historic times in the Middle East, India and China (but not in the New World) links the process with the presence of recently-domesticated animals – cows, pigs, horses, sheep, dogs, cats, chickens – in, or near, the living quarters of humankind. The proximity of beasts and humans, over time, encouraged the disease-bearing parasites of particular animals to try their luck with humans. Then, as now, the disease agents bred rapidly, producing thousands of offspring. Those few progeny that happened to have the ability to reproduce themselves in humans, in turn, produced thousands of progeny, genetically almost like themselves. With this evolutionary process (first hinted at by Charles Darwin in 1859 in his *On the Origin of Species*), a new human affliction had come into being.

A standard example of species-jumping is cow-pox which, through the processes of evolution, perhaps somewhere in Asia, converted itself from a bovine disease into various forms of smallpox, a viral disease. As it happened, the form of smallpox found in the Middle East in the twelfth century of our era was not (according to a Muslim medical writer of the time) particularly dangerous. Many children suffered from it, but most survived and acquired immunity from further attacks of the disease. But in some parts of the world, such as the Americas after 1518, or Sweden in the early eighteenth century, smallpox was a major disease killer.

Measles, another major killer viral disease in the Americas after the arrival of Columbus in 1492, may originally have been a disease of fowl which, when domesticated in India as chickens (that fluttered in and out of peasants' huts), jumped species and became a human disease. In chicken-less parts of the world, such as Ancient Egypt before 332 BCE when it was brought within the empire created by Alexander the Great, measles was apparently unknown.

A decisive element in the evolution of several of the leading infectious diseases in the Old World, and the apparent complete absence of these diseases in the New World on the eve of sustained European colonization after 1492 (and hence the disastrous absence of disease immunity among New World peoples) does not appear to be related to the density of human population as earlier medical historians thought. Indeed, it is now known that on the eve of the Spanish conquest in 1519, Tenochtitlán, the capital city of the Aztec state (now buried under Mexico City) was far larger – by a factor of 3 – than was any city in west Europe. The old thesis of urbanization – as the distinguishing characteristic of Europe – must thus be rejected.

Instead, the key difference between New World cities, towns and villages and Old World settlements was the almost complete absence of domesticated animals (other than dogs) in the New World. Ironically, it now seems that the world's first ancestral horses and camels and perhaps other largish mammals had first evolved in the New World (and then migrated west to Asia). However, it seems that by around 13,000 years ago, members of the so-called Clovis culture – descendants of Asian immigrants to the New World who are hypothesized to have walked most of the way from Asia by way of what is now the Bering Straits separating Alaska from Siberia – had slaughtered the horses and camels they found in the New World, for food. With the death of the last New World large mammals with which humankind might have come into close contact, through domestication, the opportunity for species-transfer between animal-borne disease agents and humans disappeared.

The immediate consequence was a New World which was innocent of most of the infectious diseases which had evolved in EurAsia and Africa in the years since rising sea levels had closed off ready migration between the Old World and the New by two-legged and four-legged mammals. But, as we will see in Chapter 7, absence of immunities to Old World diseases led to the near extinction of the peoples of the New World in the years after 1492, when the man from Genoa – Columbus – came among them.

Surviving evidence does not suggest that the Danish, Norse and Gotlandish survivors of abortive settlement in Greenland (tenth–fourteenth centuries) who briefly established trading missions in Labrador and the Great Lakes region in North America in the early 1360s, brought with them any major infectious diseases which remained permanently in place. The regions through which the fourteenth-century Scandinavian traders had travelled were still heavily populated by smallpox-free and measles-free First Americans when they were next observed by Europeans, in the seventeenth and early eighteenth centuries.

Some definitions and sources of information

The biological peculiarities of humankind that impact on the way they might be affected by any specific disease have only recently been of interest to medical scientists. With respect to the disease histories of past populations, it is still too early to draw large conclusions from the small number of DNA and RNA tests that have been made on the long-buried remains of earlier populations (for instance, mummified Egyptians and mummified Peruvians). In the meantime, while awaiting results from the study of large numbers of representative samples from past populations, we have to admit that the depth of time covered in the biological source material currently at our disposal remains somewhat limited.

On the other hand, if we turn to the second attribute of humankind, humans as bearers of culture, we will find that it has left a written record which in some of the more fortunate parts of the world (as in Egypt) extends back for 5,000 years (see Chapter 2). In dealing with written and archae-ological ancient sources, specialists of course now realize that it is dangerous for them to generalize from what they (the specialists) perceive to be the attitudes of a particular people at a particular point in time. They know, for example, that neighboring peoples (the Other) may have thought quite differently about the same (biologically identical) disease phenomena that were troubling the people the archaeologist is investigating.

Indeed, until relatively recently, ordinary humans identified almost entirely with their own known world of lived experience. This world included little more than their own village, the neighboring villages from which they might take spouses, and the nearest market town or center of princely authority. Beyond that (and the air space immediately above it), lay the unknown, inhabited by strange beings and evil forces.

One of the more useful insights to come out of social history in the 1970s (social history was a sub-discipline of history which analyzed such things as the space of the village) was that most of the written sources left by earlier European societies were composed by priests and other members of the literate elite at the bequest of, and for the benefit of, that society's ruling elite. Attitudes toward disease and what constituted good and evil were, in large measure, determined by the socio-economic biases of the author and his patrons. These attitudes might not be the same as those of ordinary unlettered peoples. For example, in those societies (China and India *c.* 1000 CE) which supported a professional (fee-collecting) medical estab-lishment, ordinary unlettered people would not expect to have access to professionals' store of knowledge. In those societies, high-status medical men were kept in existence largely to serve the elite.

Here, a word or two more about terminology. Used in the phrase, "humans as bearers of culture," the word "culture" refers to the commonly-shared assumptions, prejudices and opinions which adult people in a culture-group taught their children, which they, in turn, assimilated and mulled over as they grew up and, in time, submitted to a reality check. If the teachings of parents and community elders (handed down 20 or 30 years previously) still seemed to be relevant to their own world of perceived reality (and provided satisfactory answers to questions about who they were, who their ancestors were, and why), the second generation of adults would remember them and, in turn, would transmit them to their own children. But if the old teachings no longer seemed relevant they would be forgotten and so fall into oblivion.

In other words, cultures change over time, just as disease types change over time. Thus it is less than helpful to use the term, "traditional culture." The term itself was coined in the nineteenth century by European anthropologists in the employ of Imperial governments who wanted to prove that the Non-western people they had absorbed into their empire were simple-minded folk unchanged since "time immemorial" whom Western imperialists had to teach how to be "modern." In short, not only does the term "traditional culture" lack meaningful explanatory value, it is also highly charged politically. Accordingly, other than trotting it out to demonstrate the mind-set characteristic of empire builders, it should no longer be used.

In pedantic usage, it has also been claimed that there is a basic difference between the word "disease" and the words "illness" or "sickness." "Disease" as in "disease agent" is the infecting *entity* which comes in from the outside to impact upon a victim. As far as the word "illness" is concerned, a victim falls "ill" and feels sick. Yet in general parlance the distinction is often blurred: a sick person feels the opposite of healthy or "at ease" and instead feels "dis-ease."

In such matters, those who live in the West or in middle-class urban enclaves in the Non-west (in global terms, the fortunate few – the 15 percent) have to make a determined effort to grasp the grimness of past reality for most of humankind. In non-privileged, non-modern societies, most people in times past were malnourished, inadequately clothed against the elements, unwashed and filthy, living with insect parasites in over-crowded hovels. However, they had no reason to assume that this condition was not the normal lot of humankind. They knew of no one whose standard of living and life-expectations were dissimilar to their own.

In these circumstances, "ill-health" (as recorded, for example, in court-room testimony in seventeenth-century Naples) very often simply meant that one was too incapacitated to carry on working in the fields or in the shop. It did not mean that one woke up feeling slightly off-color, knowing (as moderns do) that the medicine cabinet was full of pills, any one of which – according to advertisements on television – would make one feel better. Thus, in contrast to the situation in the present day West where good health, according to advertisers and marketeers, is supposed to be the norm, in the world we have lost, feeling somewhat off-color (or worse) was the standard condition.

For this reason, the demographic materials preserved from earlier record-keeping societies (population surveys, baptism records and so on) make grim reading. Though detailed analysis of the records of particular administrative units (such as parishes) show there were important shifts one way or the other, in general one finds high (in modern Western terms) infant and child mortality rates (perhaps 200 or 400 per 1,000 live births per year). These went along with an average life expectancy for adults that was very short. Fewer than one in three of the infants born survived long enough to marry and have children of their own. One in three women died in the course of attempting to give birth. In less fortunate regions (where nature and the local war lords were harsh), average life expectancy at birth hovered around the age of 25. In regions better provided with a regular food supply and a modicum of law and order it might hover between 35 and 40. Globally, death was a constant companion.

Pluralism of cures and of perceived causal factors of disease

Nowadays it is said that, when feeling sick, 20 percent of the people of England and 40 percent of the people of North America (these are of course both "developed societies") turn for relief either entirely to alternative medicine or supplement biomedicine by having some recourse to alternative medicine. This is an example of medical pluralism. Yet, for the historian, when dealing with times past (when there were no "developed societies" as we understand the term), the concept "pluralism" also applies to the great range of answers which people trotted out to explain what had caused their own, their loved ones' or their enemy's mortal illness.

As bearers of culture, human beings in earlier times were limited in their range of supposed causal agents by the boundaries of their own culture. (This was of course before TV and other global information systems came into being and supposedly enlarged users' perceptions). Medieval and early modern Christians thus believed in the very real existence of a benevolent God and of a malevolent Devil. Accordingly, they might see an epidemic disease that struck their city as being sent down by God to punish them for their corporate sins, for instance, for allowing female and male prostitutes to openly solicit passers-by. Alternatively, medieval Christians might hold that the bubonic plague or leprosy currently wreaking havoc in their cities was caused by resident Jewish folk who, it was thought, were going around poisoning the town wells.

In the Christian West after the eleventh century, another explanation was that a particular illness had been sent in by a worshipper of the Devil who had renounced God, a witch. This sort of explanation had a long future ahead of it. As recently as 1903 notices were found in *The Times* (London) about local English people claiming they had been overlooked and made ill by a neighborhood witch. In rural Norway, as late as the 1980s, accusations of witchcraft were still being made, though they were not acted upon by magistrates or others in authority.

As the pioneer colonial anthropologist, E. E. Evans-Pritchard, pointed out long ago in his study of witchcraft among the Azande (Sudan), a witchcraft accusation provided an answer to the basic question "why me?" which modern medical science generally failed to address. The accuser fell sick, yet many other people in the community were not struck down by the same illness, even though their life-style, diet and so on were identical. According to this mind-set, the sick person had obviously been singled out and bewitched. This explanation provided a human causal agent who very possibly could be dealt with in one way or another. This sort of explanation was far more emotionally satisfying than one which held that one was struck down sick by some impersonal force – chance or fate – against which effective action was impossible.

To take a more specific example, in and around my former university city in Yorubaland in West Africa, in the last century, explanations about the cause of disease remained richly pluralistic. In addition to straightforward natural causation (a hammer hitting a blacksmith's fingernail, causing an infection), and accusations of witchcraft against a known person, there was also the possibility that the sick person was at odds with a recently dead ancestor, and that the ancestor was sending down illness as punishment. This causal relationship might well go beyond the single ancestor, and involve the whole of the sick-person's social relationship with an important element of the community. To sort through this web of complexities, a traditional healer was generally called in.

In early modern Europe, among members of the elite as well as among the populace at large, ideas about disease being caused by witches or by poison-spreading enemies of God sometimes co-existed with the notion that disease was caused by happenings among the stars and planets. Astrology was a learned art which, in theory, dated back to Ancient Sumer, but which, in practice, underwent periodic lapses, followed by rebirths and renewals. It was based on the notion that there was a direct connection between individual humankind (particularly the fee-paying wealthy) and the movements of the heavenly bodies. It held that if one knew the precise locations of relevant heavenly bodies at the moment of one's birth, accurate predictions could be made about one's life chances, marriage and final end.

Going beyond the individual level, in the Middle Ages, university-educated medical doctors sometimes linked disease happenings which affected whole societies to happenings among the planets. Thus, when the bubonic plague (the Black Death) first hit northern Europe in 1348, court physicians informed the King of France that the plague had come into being with the conjunction of the planets Saturn, Jupiter and Mars on 14 March 1345 and that this had caused the heating of the air which, in turn, caused a miasma which itself caused the buboes of plague to break out on the bodies of sufferers. It will be noticed that this causal explanation contained two elements. One was directly derived from astrology, and the other – which posited a miasma – was derived from Hippocrates (the fifth–fourth-century BCE Greek father of medicine) by way of later translators and simplifiers.

In the book that follows I will often be referring to the triangle of healing. The three elements involved are (1) the disease itself (whether actual pathogen or imagined entity); (2) the sick person who looks for advice to an expert (variously defined); and (3) the curer. The skills the curer displayed were necessarily accepted as legitimate in his/her own culture (otherwise the curer would go out of business). These skills often included an understanding of the web of local social relationships among the living (and the recent dead) which the sick person has inadvertently run afoul of. The curer would know how to reincorporate this person into an acceptable role, restoring social harmony, thus "curing" the sick person (which might merely mean enabling him or her to bear pain without further complaint or sense of guilt).

Plan of the book

In order to meaningfully discuss disease and medicine in world history, and to avoid the pitfalls found in old-style Whiggish texts, special stress must be placed on differences, disconnectedness and discontinuities. This approach permits us to appreciate the essential uniqueness and intellectual integrity of each of the cultural-social groupings dealt with in this book.

On this issue, it is well to remember that the processes of "globalization" which seem so overwhelmingly important to us today did not, in fact, begin to get under way until after 1500: (in retrospect, the early Portuguese, Spanish and Genoese navigators can be seen as pioneer "globalizers"). As late as 1800 or 1840, among people living in great Non-western civilizational centers such as China or South Asia, the concept of "globalization" (as present-day Western readers understand the term) would have been utterly meaningless: it was irrelevant to lived experience.

I have deliberately chosen the order in which the societies I examine are presented. Following on from my discussion of extinct societies – ancient Egypt and the pre-conquest Americas (Chapter 2) – I present some of the dead-end ideas found in ancient Greece which the ancient Greeks themselves abandoned. I also present some of the more important ideas which successor societies claimed to have inherited from ancient Greece. These "remembered" ideas – which constituted only a fragment of the medical lore of ancient

Greece – became the basis of the so called "Great Tradition." This Great Tradition would form an important part of what passed for learned (as opposed to household and folk) medicine in the imperial city of Rome itself and, after the fall of the Roman Empire in the West, in the Roman/Byzantine imperial capital in the East, Constantinople.

However as will be seen, with the decay of secular learning on the northern side of the Mediterranean (and the triumph of religious obscurantism in Byzantium), the Greco-Roman medical legacy would have been lost forever had it not been rescued from oblivion by Muslim writers living to the south and east of that inland sea. In Chapter 4, I will examine the largely reworked "Great Tradition" as it emerged from the hands of Muslim writers from the seventh century onwards. In its new forms it was synthesized and, in later centuries, transferred to new centers of learning in Italy and across the Alps. Thus was preserved what is arguably the oldest of the world's great medical traditions.

Following on from the Middle East and its updated Greek tradition (with Persian, Arabian and Egyptian additions), I next turn to ancient India. As will be seen, it is extremely difficult to come up with a single, generally accepted date which marks the beginning of the traditions which came together to form Ayurvédic medicine sometime early in the present era (CE). In any case, Ayurvédic medicine had ceased being receptive to outside influences (leading to system modification) some centuries before Chinese medicine did so. By introducing China's medical systems in the chapter following that on India, I am able to place a Chinese attempt at assimilation of Indian medical ideas in an appropriate chronological context.

The order in which the last four chapters are presented requires little explanation. I begin with the globalization of the diseases of the Old World (the EurAsian continent and Africa) after 1450 (Chapter 7) and then turn (in Chapter 8) to a brief examination of medical ideas and disease crises in western Europe between the recovery of the Great Tradition (c. 1050) and 1840. Then, in Chapter 9, I examine the break with the Great Tradition, and the birth of modern medicine in the German lands (united into a single country in 1871). I also examine the somewhat quirky forms of medical modernization developed in Great Britain in the last half of the nineteenth century and then go on to see what became of these ideas in British-ruled India after 1868.

In the final chapter (Chapter 10), I look at the present-day situation as it emerged after 1943 when Western medical science finally developed the miracle drugs which alone seemed able to actually cure a whole host of infectious diseases. These developments led, in our own time, to the creation of aging populations in the West, quantitatively and qualitatively different from any population which had existed anywhere in the world in the past.

In Chapter 10 I also explore why two-fifths of the people in the present-day world do not have access to modern Western medicine, even though most of them desperately want it and would use it if they could. We find that since these unfortunate people have incomes of less than $2.00 a day, they simply cannot afford Western medicine or Western medical care. On this issue, those of the world's poor who live in the Non-west also come up against the mindsets of Western finance officials. Among these gentlemen's immediate predecessors and prototypes – the colonial elites in charge of British India – these mindsets first became established in coherent form in the late 1860s. Since that time there has been no appreciable change in attitudes. This is one of the more unfortunate *continuities* in the long-term global history of medicine and disease.

Further reading

For Africa, key insights into the plurality of medical systems and explanations are found in: Steven Feierman and John Janzen (eds), *The Social Basis of Health & Healing in Africa* (University of California Press, 1992). For the findings of social history from a Non-western perspective: Sheldon Watts, *A Social History of Western Europe, 1450–1720* (London: Hutchinson University Library for Africa, 1984). For introductory essays on the world's various medical systems in times past, see those by Murray Last and others in W. F. Bynum and Roy Porter (eds), *Companion Encyclopedia of the History of Medicine* (London: Routledge, 1993). On the newness of modern biomedicine see: Andrew Cunningham, Perry Williams (eds), *The Laboratory Revolution in Medicine* (Cambridge University Press, 1992).

Chapter 2

Before the advent of acute epidemic diseases. Pharaonic Egypt and the pre-conquest New World

Extinct societies

Introduction

In this chapter we consider long-dead societies which had no experience with acute epidemic diseases such as cholera, bubonic plague, measles and smallpox, or with debilitating, slow working, ultimately lethal diseases such as syphilis or leprosy. We first look at the situation in ancient Egypt under its pharaohs (3100–525 BCE). Then we briefly examine some aspects of the situation in the New World just before 1492 CE, on the eve of European conquest and permanent settlement. Our foray in the New World will focus only on literate (or record-keeping), now extinct, societies in Central and South America. Later (in Chapter 7) we will widen our view to include societies in North America.

Information sources: ancient Egypt

Pharaonic Egypt provides us with the world's earliest sizeable corpus of evidence about people's health status, about medical ideas, and about the treatments doctors might have used. This unique situation is due to three circumstances.

First, it is due to the special qualities of ancient Egypt's natural environment. Ninety-five percent of the country was desert (90 percent remains desert today). Arable farming was confined to the banks of the Nile, the great river which cuts through the desert and runs from south to north. Given this natural environment, survival of the actual physical remains of large numbers of dead people (marvelous sources of medical information) is due to ancient Egyptian unwillingness to cremate their dead. Instead of incinerating the corpses of ordinary people, they generally buried them in the sands. Higher status people, after death, often were embalmed (converted into mummies) and buried in dry, reasonably secure stone-built tombs. Both forms of burial ensured the preservation of corpses into modern times.

Also contributing greatly to our knowledge was the literacy of ancient Egyptian priestly castes. Writing on papyrus (tightly woven leaves) enabled them to create permanent records. These thousands of papyri (records written in hieroglyphics – the oldest still surviving dates from 1820 BCE), have proved to be immensely helpful, even if they are at times misleading. Unintelligible for nearly 1,400 years after the death of the last indigenous person who could read them (around 420 CE), Egyptian hieroglyphs were not again read until 1822, when the Frenchman, J. F. Champollion, made his intuitive breakthrough into comprehension.

Though the papyri surviving to our own day (many of which are copies of documents 1,000 years older) tell us a great deal about what seems to be medical matters, unfortunately many important hieroglyphic symbols dealing with diseases and body parts are found *only* in the medical papyri. This means that their meaning cannot be checked with reference to other sources and that meaning has to be inferred from the "medical" context. To "infer" necessarily means being "subjective" and coming up with a meaning that *may* not have been what the Ancients meant. Indeed, in-depth studies currently being carried out on hieroglyphics show that the mind-set of the ancient Egyptians was utterly unlike any mind-set known in the world today. This means that at best, today's interpretations of the medical papyri can only be regarded as provisional.

In addition to these written records (the medical papyri) and the actual bodies of the dead, ancient artists and workmen sculpted, carved and painted thousands of representations of Egyptian people (and their gods) engaged in ordinary everyday activities. Some of these carvings are of dwarfs or hunchbacks. For example, one 12-inch-high wooden statue from Saqqarah dating from *c.* 2500 BCE, now on display at the Egyptian Museum, portrays a man who may have been suffering from Potts disease (spinal tuberculosis). Representations such as this suggest that the ancient Egyptians sympathized with those less fortunate than themselves, presumably just as we do today.

Yet this sense of familiarity with ancient Egyptians should be resisted. In the interest of objective understanding, they must be regarded as alien peoples whose thought processes, conceptions of earthly reality, and of the supernatural were entirely different from our own. They are a quintessential Other.

It is in this context that we point out that the gullible Greek traveler/ historian, Herodotus, visited Egypt around 450 BCE. This was some seventy-five years after the Persians had conquered the country and wrought great havoc in the north (destroying temple complexes and whole cities). At the time of Herodotus's visit, Egypt was well past its days of glory and was still nominally under Persian rule.

Herodotus (sometimes called the Father of History) wrote a famous account of his Egyptian travels and gave detailed descriptions (including things of medical interest) of what he claimed he had seen. However, many experts are convinced that Herodotus didn't actually go much further south than the (now ruined, largely unexcavated) temple complex at Heliopolis (10 miles north of the center of modern Cairo).

What with one thing and another, Herodotus came away with many strange ideas about Egypt. Sometimes called the "father of lies," the father of history did, however, write about some topics (i.e. infant mortality rates) which no native Egyptian scribe, that we know of, mentioned. He also claimed that the Egyptian medical profession was divided into various specialties – dentistry, surgery and so on. Because he provided us with clues such as these (even if they have not been substantiated), Herodotus cannot be completely ignored.

Ancient Egyptian ideas about the body

The ancient Egyptians thought that humans were born healthy. If people fell ill, it was because something foreign (spiritual or material) had entered their bodies. In other ways as well Egyptian ideas were, shall we say, "interesting." For a start, they believed that the human *brain* did not have any particularly useful function. Thus, when preparing the body of a dead person for mummification, the embalmer drew out the brain matter through a tube forced through the nose into the skull. The brain-pulp was then discarded, being seen as of no importance for the well-being of the dead in the afterlife.

Yet, four other bodily organs (seen as necessary in the life to come) were carefully preserved, each placed in a Canopic jar left near the mummified corpse. These jars held the liver, the lungs, the stomach and the intestines. The heart, seen as essential for life (and from which the spirit of the departed acquired the energy needed to gather up his other body parts before going out visiting) was left in the mummy. Considered to be the most important of all the bodily organs, the heart was also regarded as the seat of the human soul (the *ba*).

In all this it is important to point out that ancient Egyptian medical doctors (claiming professional competence to cure some of the diseases suffered by living people) seem to have held embalmers in contempt. This socially sanctioned prejudice against the specialists who created mummies meant that physicians were not in a position to gain new insights from the category of people who had the best hands-on knowledge of some parts of the human anatomy. This communication failure may, in part, explain the gaps in medical men's knowledge of human anatomy. A fuller explanation however would have to point out that after the early centuries (pre-dynastic and Old Kingdom to 2181 BCE) and perhaps not even then, priest-doctors and apprentice doctors were not particularly interested in actual *human* anatomy, as opposed to anatomy as *metaphor*.

At no time in their long history did the ancient Egyptians have a clear idea about the circulatory system (veins and arteries) that carries blood to all parts of the body and back again to the heart. Indeed, they seem not to have had separate words for veins and arteries. Instead, they thought in terms of an imaginary set of channels (for which they had the special word *M-T-W*) which connected the heart with other organs of the body and ended up at, or near, the anus. This imagined set of vessels carried away *W-H-D-W*, the rot or pollution, which they regarded as the secondary causal agent of disease. For them the primary cause was either a material force (such as a snake bite) or a spiritual force coming in from the outside.

Close reading of the three medical papyri which deal with gynecological matters does not suggest that the ancient Egyptians had any understanding of the role of a women's egg. As we now know, the egg when fertilized by a man's sperm develops into a fetus. In the making of this end-result, an unborn human baby, the woman's contribution is no less vital than that made by the man.

The Egyptians did realize that a man's testicles were important in the production of sperm. Sperm was regarded as a positive, life-giving force (we will see parallels to this in ancient Chinese medical ideas). In Egyptian mythology, the creator God, Atun, had produced the sky gods Shu (air) and Tefnut (moisture, clouds, water) from his sperm. These gods had produced other gods who, in turn, had created humankind. Life-affirming in these and other ways, a man's sperm was also seen as a destructive force. A sick Egyptian male might dream that he had been poisoned and made ill by an enemy's sperm. From this it followed that homosexual acts (between human males) were generally regarded as unspeakably evil: this rule however did not hold for the gods.

Before the conquest of Egypt by the Greek-speaking armies of Alexander the Great in 332 BCE, the ancient Egyptians had no experience with mass-killing, acute infectious diseases. They had no bubonic plague, no cholera, no measles and probably no locally based endemic malaria. This last disease deserves further comment.

In Egypt's medical papyri (which pre-date the Greek Conquest) there is no reference to anything resembling malaria with its alarmingly rapid rise and fall of temperatures, its debilitating effects and high mortality. In Greece itself (from whence Alexander the Great later came), Hesiod, the author of "Life and Days" in the mid-sixth century BCE, likewise made no mention of anything which could be construed to be malaria, even though he went on at great length about the innumerable hardships faced by Greek farmers in the "age of iron" which he claimed had followed after the (mythic) "age of gold." But by the time of Hippocrates (the alleged father of Western medicine) who lived and wrote only one year before the birth of Alexander the Great (Hippocrates died *c.* 357 BCE; Alexander was born 356 BCE), malaria was clearly well established in mainland Greece and the isles. From thence, it is not unlikely that it was carried by peripatetic Hellenistic Greeks to Egypt where it became endemic.

The situation regarding smallpox remains ambivalent. Despite a recent claim that the mummy of Rameses V (died 1156 BCE, now on display in the

Egyptian Museum) shows the pustules of smallpox, there are no similar mummies and no mention of any mass-death of people from disease as there would have been had epidemics of smallpox actually swept over ancient Egypt. As we will see in Chapter 7 (when we examine the murderous impact of smallpox in the Americas after 1518), in times past, isolated, single cases of a violently infectious disease like smallpox (or measles) are unlikely to have occurred. And in a highly literate country like Egypt it is most unlikely that region-wide epidemics which killed off half of the population every twenty-five or thirty years would not have been recorded, either in writing or in sculpture. Thus, it is not surprising that ancient Egyptian experts in formal medicine had no words for, or – so it seems – knowledge of, contagious or infectious diseases.

The role of formal medicine in pharaoh's palace and in temples

The fifteen most important, still extant, medical papyri from ancient Egypt include the Edwin Smith (from 1550 BCE), the Ebers (from 1500 BCE), the Brooklyn (from 300 BCE), and the Chester Beatty VI (from 1200 BCE). From internal evidence it has been shown that these papyri are actually copies of papyri originally made 500 or 1,000 years earlier. The inferred existence of the earlier papyri (dating back to the Old Kingdom) enables us to claim that the ancient Egyptian system of formal medicine (for the elite) was the first of its kind in the world.

Established in the pre-literate, pre-dynastic period and in the Old Kingdom (2613–2181 BCE), the standard Egyptian pattern of clinical practice apparently remained in use in pharaoh's land for thousands of years. According to the formula, a doctor would examine the patient, asking set questions to find out what the problem was. He (gender deliberate) would then arrive at his prognosis; the disease was such and such. The doctor then either recommended a cure, or confessed that the situation was hopeless.

Several points emerge from what I have just said. First, it is known that there actually *was* a woman doctor (or overseer of doctors) named Peseshet sometime in the period 2494 to 2181 BCE. However, no other group of women is known to have served as doctors until after the Greek conquest in 323 BCE.

Paralleling the male domination of the formal medical sector for 1,800 years, was the absence of any special word for "midwife" in the ancient Egyptian language. Babies obviously were born, but apparently no earthly specialists were called in as attendants. Aside from help from the frog goddess Heqet (recorded as having come down in disguise to serve as birth attendant), ordinary village women apparently did what was necessary to comfort the woman in labor on her special birthing chair.

Another interesting point is that the long-term flow of Egyptian medicine ran quite contrary to what modern research scientists writing in 1910 (such as Ronald Ross) assumed must have been the case. Ross was convinced that the field of medicine had always moved from "magic" to "science." However, detailed recent research strongly suggests that pre-dynastic and Old Kingdom medicine (3100–2181 BCE) was more solidly based on empirical experience and reason (establishing a correlation between physical cause and physical effect) than was medicine in the late New Kingdom and the Persian periods. In short, the order of movement in real-world Egypt seems to have been *from* science *to* magic.

Various suggestions have been made for why this happened. As there are no written sources telling us how a young man learned to be a physician, it would appear that potential entrants to the profession often trained as priests. This training in temples dedicated to the goddess Sekhmet (the lion-headed daughter of Re) equipped them to serve as guardians of tradition: they would not be open to new ideas. Young men who trained as apprentices to an established doctor but never became priests doubtless would not have had the social clout needed to counter the dead weight of priestly tradition.

Already by the end of the Old Kingdom (2181 BCE) the Egyptian elite had become intensely conservative. Priest-doctors, when looking across from old Memphis (the pharaonic capital) to the west bank of the Nile, would cast their eyes on the Great Pyramids and the walls surrounding the Sphinx. These vast monuments, put up more than 500 years before their own time, were a clear demonstration to priest-doctor observers that their ancestors had been intellectual giants. From this it seemed to follow that the truths revealed to these ancestors (including medical truths) must be accepted and cherished.

In any case, the holy men who served as medical attendants on Pharaoh and his courtiers seemingly achieved these positions of trust not so much because they were able to cure any disease by the application of anything other than common sense (tender loving care, soothing food, and, as the phrase went, recommending "staying in dock") but because they could call to mind and recite the appropriate ancient traditions. As we will see, this in fact was the case in nearly all societies until almost our own time (radical change only came with the advent of antibiotics and other miracle drugs in the 1940s and 1950s).

In ancient Egypt, the cherishing of tradition was demonstrated by the career of Imhotep. As a living being, Imhotep was the chancellor and first secretary of Zozer, the second pharaoh in the third dynasty (2667–2648 BCE). Among his achievements, Imhotep designed and oversaw the building of the Step Pyramid, the oldest still-surviving large stone building in the world. The construction of this mighty pyramid was obviously a great achievement: Imhotep was recognized to be an inspired genius. Within 100 years of his death, pilgrims in search of wisdom had begun to visit his tomb.

During Imhotep's lifetime and for hundreds of years thereafter, no one suggested that he had had anything to do with the practice of medicine.

Then, more than 2,000 years (400 generations) after his death, following the Persian conquest (525 BCE) when it was obvious that things were going badly wrong, nostalgic Egyptians noticed that they had no special god of medicine. They also noticed that the Greeks (the up and coming cultural grouping across the Mediterranean) did have a god of medicine (Asclepius; see Chapter 3). So, as representatives of the oldest culture in the region, the Egyptians decided that they must follow the Greek precedent. Accordingly, Imhotep (already revered as a god of wisdom) came to be revered as a God of Medicine.

Somewhat similar are the claims that there was progress in surgery in ancient Egypt. In the tomb near Saqqarah of Qar, pharaoh's chief surgeon, of around 2300 BCE, a set of 30 scalpels and tweezers has recently (mid-2001) been found. Nothing like them from any later period has (to date) been discovered, even though scalpels and tweezers are mentioned in some Middle Kingdom papyri. This suggests that practical surgery may indeed have been performed in the early years of the pharaonic period, but that it was then all but given up, probably because most surgeons' patients died.

Here it is appropriate point out that the Hellenistic Greek founders of the great schools at Alexandria (after 332 BCE) purposely excluded Egyptian students (the anachronistic word, apartheid, best explains the situation). When, a few years later, Greek physicians such as Herophilus (around 330–260/250 BCE) came to Alexandria to practice medicine, they denounced the whole medical lore of ancient Egypt, saying it was rubbish. Going further, Herophilus became famous for conducting public anatomy lessons on still-living, screaming, Egyptian convicts donated to him by the sophisticated Greek Ptolemaic ruler of Egypt (see Chapter 3).

The role of Egyptian medicine in everyday life

Graveyards of ancient Egyptians, knowledgeably excavated, provide useful evidence about the diseases from which these people suffered and the success or otherwise of medical interventions. Thus far, the largest excavation to have been published (entered into the public domain) was made when 6,000 bodies had to be hastily moved from low-lying ground near the first Aswan Dam. Though the sophisticated techniques for examining the dead developed since then (X-rays, DNA testing, RNA testing, etc.) were obviously not used, nevertheless the 6,000 dead managed to tell us several things.

First, they partially address the issue of ancient Egyptian dental skills. Herodotus in writing his observations of Egypt in 450 BCE, claimed that dentists were a separate branch of medicine. However, among the 6,000 dead at Aswan, there was no evidence of anyone having had their teeth *successfully* repaired. Perhaps this was simply because Aswan was so far distant from capital cities with their dental experts. But until such time as new work on mummies and corpses buried near capital cities proves otherwise, we can assume that specialized dental work was beyond the capabilities of the ancient Egyptians. This was an unfortunate gap.

Because of the nature of the impurities in the foods they ate, many ancient Egyptians over the age of twenty-five had problems with their teeth. The principal foodstuff was one of several early forms of wheat, barley or rye. All these had to be ground up for flour for the making of bread. This is where the problem lay. During milling operations, the grinding stones released small particles of stone. These bits of stone (together with sand blown in from the surrounding desert) found their way into the bread. Chewed on over the years, these bits of stony grit wore through the enamel on people's teeth, exposing the blood vessels, and nerves and pulp at the center of the tooth. Though we have nothing resembling statistics from ancient Egypt, we can assume that mortality rates from infected teeth must have been high.

Before we move on from teeth, we should first notice that the ancient Egyptian diet did not contain great quantities of honey or other sweet things. This meant that their teeth were not rotted out by sugar, even though they were likely to be ground down by sand. Excavations of grave-yards show that this situation changed for the worse after the coming of the Persians in 525 BCE when, among the locals, the foreign taste for sweets caught on.

Used in another way however, honey was an important constituent part of Egyptian medicine. It seems to have been noticed back in pre-dynastic and Old Kingdom times that honey applied to a wound prevented the development of gangrene, and with it the need for amputating the affected limb. Though not yet subjected to statistical confirmation, among existing mummies, a largish number seem to have nicely recovered from fractured bones. This suggests that, in addition to knowing about splints for broken arms or legs, the ancient Egyptian had come to realize that petrification of the member (modern gangrene) could be prevented by liberal applications of honey on the wound.

Recent excavation work in the workers' cemetery in Saqqarah (near the Step Pyramid) and from Dahkhla Oasis in the Western Desert have shown that neck and spinal injuries caused by carrying heavy weights on the head for long distances were a major cause of death among workers in these places. The human frame was not built for this sort of usage.

This raises the more general issue of life expectancy among the one and a quarter to two million people living at any one time in Old Kingdom Egypt and the seven million living in Egypt on the eve of the Greek conquest. Recent studies of dried corpses from both eras suggest that among the population who survived the first 12 months after the trauma of birth, life expectancy for males ranged between 30 and 39 (that for women was five years less). This is about the same as found before 1900 CE in some of the more fortunate parts of *rural* western Europe; before 1900, life expectancy for youthful male rural migrants coming into urban places such as London or Frankfurt-am-Main was much shorter (25 to 30).

Modern techniques do show that a sizeable number of ancient Egyptians lived well beyond the average life span. Rameses II, for example (reigned 1304–1237 BCE) kept himself in fine form by siring several hundred children and died at the age of 94; study of his mummified remains confirms that he was indeed very old at the time of his death. Pepi II (sixth dynasty), according to standard calculations, reigned for more than 90 years. Even if this figure is cut in half (as revisionists claim is necessary) a reign of 45 years is still impressive.

In the absence of major acute infectious diseases, what then were the principal causes of death in ancient Egypt? We have already mentioned infected teeth, broken bones and neck and spinal injuries. We must also mention famine. During periods when the Nile failed to rise to its usual level during the annual inundation, grain and other food reserves may have been used up, leading to starvation. Hydrological historians tell us that famines may have been common during the long run of disastrous years known to us as the First Intermediate Period (c. 2181 to 2050 BCE) and the Second Intermediate Period (c. 1786 to 1567 BCE). During these years, Nile inundations fell well below their Old Kingdom norms.

In addition to death from starvation or a famine-related disease, countless ordinary people who cultivated crops near the Nile were pulled into the river and eaten by crocodiles. Snake bites and bites from scorpions were also a major cause of death. During the long Egyptian centuries, snake bite was seen as something sent in from the outside, against which all medical remedies were useless. Only a miracle (using a special anti-snake stone carving over which water was poured: the water was then drunk) could save the afflicted. More than two dozen of these Horus stelae as they are called, some 2–3 inches high and portable, some much larger and not portable, are currently on display at the Egyptian Museum in Cairo.

Yet suggestive of a certain degree of intellectual vitality, according to the Brooklyn papyrus (300 BCE), written just before or just after the Greek conquest, priestly medical doctors had managed to identify more than 20 different biting snakes (some lethal, some not so) and had devised specific cures for each sort of bite. Yet, it cannot be expected that these mystic cures (sanctified herbs and drugs locked away in the confines of a temple dedicated to the goddess Sekhmet) would be of much relevance to the needs of a peasant cultivator or herdsman who was bitten many miles distant from formal medical assistance.

Among ordinary people there were also several debilitating diseases. Undoubtedly, first in importance as cause of death among newborn babies and young children were water-related diarrheal diseases. Although Herodotus claimed that the Egyptians were exceptionally clean people, always bathing and washing out the simple kilt with which they covered their private parts, cleanliness did not necessarily extend to their drinking water supplies. The consumption of contaminated water during the months when the Nile was low and local water reservoirs had dried up doubtless led to annual lethal bouts of diarrheal diseases, especially among the very young.

In pharaonic Egypt, debilitation and death *might* also have been caused by the water-related parasitic disease, schistosomiasis. The parasite larva would have penetrated the skin when a person entered the Nile or the specially constructed canals and polders used to hold water for irrigation (the system known as basin irrigation). Soon after infection with *Schistosoma haematobium*, sufferers would begin to have blood in their urine. The larva matured as a worm and ultimately ended up in the liver (the filtering organ necessary for human life), but it would also be found in the kidneys, and other internal organs. Because embalmers, in the process of mummification, generally didn't reach far enough into a corpse to remove the kidneys (which in any case they may not have known about), bits of kidney surviving into the 1990s reveal that schistosomiasis *may* have been a fairly common disease. Or it may not: the examples which have been found (for instance, those at Ain Labakha in Kharga Oasis from the time of Augustus Caesar) might have been atypical. Curiously enough, in the medical papyri there is no hieroglyphic symbol which, according to modern experts, can be properly translated as meaning schistosomiasis.

One pharaoh in the Old Kingdom maintained a physician who bore the title, "shepherd of the king's anus"; perhaps others did as well. In any case, Herodotus claimed that Egyptians (when compared to his own people, the Greeks) had a particular hang-up about anal problems and were always washing out their bowels with special purges. A medical papyrus written just after the time of Rameses II (1200 BCE) contains some 41 different remedies for anal problems. Administered by priest-physicians, these ranged from incantations to soothing ointments.

In summing up this section, we must point out that by New Kingdom times (when Egyptian culture had been in existence for more than 2,100 years) formally recognized medical practice was essentially one of spiritual intervention, consisting largely of incantations by the priests of Sakhmet, officially termed "physicians." It touched hardly at all upon the lives of ordinary people.

In time of sickness, rather than looking to formal medicine, ordinary Egyptians looked to their immediate family and to local artifacts for comfort. Archaeologists have found that some of them made offerings to the little clay figures of household gods (such as Bes – a pot-bellied dwarf who was introduced to Egypt in New Kingdom times perhaps from Libya) who were thought to be interested in the welfare of humankind. Not particularly well served by their rulers' medical system, or by the irregular bounty of nature, most ordinary Egyptians were stunted folk, less than five feet two inches tall. Thus, despite the claims of New Age devotees, we should not look to the ancient Egyptians for new wisdom about the human body, or cures for physical afflictions.

Medicine in the Americas: 450 CE to 1492

Because of the accidents of history, the nature of surviving evidence, and the uneven development of the relevant scholarly disciplines in the West, at the moment we know far more about the medical lore and health conditions of the ancient Egyptians than we do about such matters among the indigenous people of South, Central, and North America on the eve of their subjugation by Europeans (beginning in 1492 CE). Let us compare what is known about demographics.

By general agreement, we know that the population of pharaonic Egypt (as it was before 525 BCE, 25 centuries ago) moved upwards from one and a quarter million to seven million. Growth seems to have been slow and steady; population never seems to have been permanently cut back by major disease disasters. By way of contrast, there is absolutely no consensus at all among those who study pre-contact New World population size.

On the one side are Euro-American scholars who cite an overall population of eight to ten million in 1491/2 (the same as that of the French hexagon at the time). On the other side are those who cite much higher figures: 75 million, or perhaps even 145 million pre-conquest New World peoples (three times more numerous than all Europeans – from Dublin to Moscow – in 1492). The huge gap between competing claims can, in part, be explained by the scarcity of surviving source materials. However, subjective factors at work in each scholar's mind must also be taken into account.

Information sources

Two cultural groupings in pre-conquest America were fully literate (the Maya and the Aztecs). Further to the south, the Incas created aides-memoire by knotting ropes in complex ways. Had great quantities of Mayan and Aztec writings extant in 1491 survived until the present, we would perhaps be in a position to know something about their diseases, medicines and general attitudes toward health. But this was not to be. In the 1560s the Spanish Christian, Diego de Landa, governor of the conquered Maya lands (in the Yucatan) deliberately incinerated whole libraries of Mayan records, seeing them as pagan nonsense. Out of thousands, only three small volumes escaped detection. Around the same time, Spanish Christians destroyed all the rope records of the Incas. Similar orgies of burning manuscripts and destroying monuments had already taken place in central Mexico, following soon after the Spanish triumph over the Aztecs in Tenochtitlán, the capital city (on 13 August 1521).

Fortunately, the knowledge-base of Central and South America was not entirely lost: some elderly New World people remained alive after the Spanish took over. It was they who served as first generation sources for oral history. As it happened, two Christian priests who went to the New World soon after the conquest (Bernardio de Sahagun, d. 1590, and Francisco de Avila, fl. 1597) decided that in order to convert New World peoples to their own true religion, it might be useful to know something about the earlier world views of the conquered peoples.

Working with aging Aztecs and youthful bi-cultural translators (who had Spanish fathers, Aztec mothers), Sahagun recorded the oral history of these people. De Avila did the same for the Incas: his work was supplemented by that of Guaman Poma, another sixteenth-century priest. Useful as the resulting compilations are, it must be stressed that Aztec and Inca oral history (recorded in Western script and eventually printed) was filtered through the minds of European priest-editors. By its very nature, this filtering led to a blurring of some of the basic differences between the ways Spanish Europeans thought about things and the ways in which New World peoples did. As a result, it is entirely likely that much that was unique to New World thought (and was known to the sixteenth-century oral history informants themselves) was forever lost.

As conventionally educated Europeans, Sahagun's and de Avila's ideas about medical matters were essentially those of Hippocrates (of ancient Greece) as revitalized by Galen (of late pagan Rome), then again revitalized by Ibn Sina (the early eleventh-century Muslim, known in the West as Avicenna) and translated into Latin for the use of Christian medical students and doctors (see Chapters 3 and 4). Let us briefly remind ourselves of these ideas. Galen's core notion (which he had obtained from certain parts of the Hippocratic Corpus) was that human health was shaped by the balance in the human body of the four humors (blood, phlegm, yellow bile and black bile). These humors corresponded to what some of the Hippocratic writers held were the four elements of external nature: earth, air, fire and water: a physician's chief task was to restore the balance among his patient's humors. It was with Galen's interpretation of Hippocrates at the back of their minds that Sahagun and Avila undertook their compilation (perhaps a better word would be "fabrication") of the medical aspects of Aztec and of Inca oral history.

Complementing these highly suspect written sources, are the skeletal remains of the small numbers of New World peoples which have already been dug up and examined. In addition, some of the mummies made up by the Incas and subordinate peoples living in the high Andes have been retrieved and studied.

Other than these two categories of sources (Spanish-filtered oral history and bodily remains) there are modern scholarly recreations of past reality which have been formulated by using the conceptual tool known as "argument by analogy." Those who use this tool work on the assumption that some of the medical ideas and practices still current among indigenous people in the high Andes are based on notions that were current long before the Spanish conquest. This presupposition is "interesting" in as much as it comes out of the same conceptual pot as the old nineteenth-century Imperial British and French notion of "native" customs unchanged "since time immemorial."

Disease types

Thus far, medical archaeologists have found no evidence that pre-contact New World peoples suffered from any of the acute infectious diseases of the Old World (smallpox, measles, cholera, malaria, bubonic plague, influenza). As we stated earlier, this was undoubtedly because animals and fowl of the kind which might be domesticated, and brought to live in close contact with humankind, were no longer found in the New World (see Chapter 1). The domesticated dogs that were there apparently did not harbor the potential disease agents which, through the process of natural selection, might jump species and create a pathogen for any of the acute infectious diseases I have mentioned.

Yet before the Spanish arrived, the western hemisphere was certainly not a disease-free paradise. Older people, of which there were only a few relative to overall population, tended to suffer from painful swelling of the joints – arthritis in one or other of its forms. In the high Andes, some people also suffered from bothersome infectious diseases carried by biting insects; their mummies show swollen skin tissues in the nose and on the face. There were also nasty single-celled creatures (amoebae) in food or drinking water which could cause diarrhea or fevers.

Then, too, there were treponema agents which caused irritating sorts of skin diseases: yaws, pinta and bejel. These agents were not transferred from one person to another through genital contact. Instead, transfer could be made (among roughhousing children for example) by rubbing an uninfected person's upper legs, arms or chest against infected skin on the face, chest, legs or arms of the yaws/pinta/bejel sufferer.

In addition to these non-venereal diseases, there might have been problems with disease agents carried in the fecal matter of lice: at the moment experts are debating whether typhus was (or was not) found in the Andes. During times of food-shortage and famine, this disease could have wrought great havoc among ill-nourished populations. However it would seem that further north, among the Aztecs, complex food distribution systems insured that most people were reasonably well fed, and accordingly would not be prone to typhus. Indeed, according to some experts, typhus was altogether unknown in the New World before the coming of the Spanish.

In the pre-contact New World, pneumonia was present, though the extent of its impact remains unknown. If it behaved as it does today, its victims were generally people who had already been debilitated by some other illness: pneumonia was simply the last of the disease conditions which sent the seriously sick to their graves.

It has been confirmed, based on tissue samples, that a form of tuberculosis was also present in the pre-contact New World. The sort found there however was a slow-acting killer which would not have resulted in dramatic numbers of deaths at any one time. In this, TB in the pre-contact New World (and in pharaonic Egypt) differed greatly from the massively contagious TB found in raw industrial cities in nineteenth-century Europe and in early twentieth-century Japan, and among the poor in the world today.

In dealing with pre-contact New World tuberculosis (as with most other diseases) a word of caution is in order. The tiny number of samples from before 1492 showing death from TB (or something like it) is far too small, relative to total population (even at its lowest estimate), to enable us to claim that TB was a widespread problem. However, it certainly became a serious problem – a mass killer – after the arrival of the Europeans.

Ideas about the universe and disease causation

When not injecting Greco-Roman-Islamic ideas about humors into their reports about the Aztecs and the Incas in the late sixteenth century, Spanish missionaries Sahagun and de Avila were perplexed to find how different these peoples' ideas were from their own. Both New World societies lived in extremely trying bio-systems over which humans had no actual physical control. They were, however, left with plenty of options in the field of metaphysics, and more especially in the sub-field known as environmental metaphysics.

Let us first turn to the Incas, dwellers in the high Andes (where temperatures might drop 60 degrees in a few minutes). Among these people, illness was thought to result if a person was out of harmony with his land and/or his family and neighbors. Complicating matters, the dis-harmony leading to illness might not be the result of the person's own wrong-doing, but of that of someone else in the family, for instance, a disloyal wife, or a disloyal husband. Causation, in short, might involve a whole complex of man/land and inter-personal relations. To discover the cause of the illness, a diviner (a specialist) would have to be called in.

Once the social cause of the illness had been sorted out, remedial actions would be taken. Remedies at the inter-personal level generally required that the wrong-doing person confess and apologize, thus restoring harmony. At that stage the sick person (who had wronged no one) might recover. Another category of actions (sometimes for the same illness) might require physical treatment. Headaches might be treated by causing bleeding on the skull or through the nose.

Alternatively, exotic drugs might be used. For people living at high altitudes (for example in the town of Cuzco at 6,000 feet) drugs might be brought up from the lowlands in the Amazon Valley, hundreds of miles away. These inter-regional transactions demonstrated the cooperative spirit and unity of people ruled (since the twelfth century) by the mighty Inca and his allies.

At the level of the individual, the Inca – and their intellectual predecessors – saw the need for the proper flow of the bodily juices and semi-liquid matter (air, blood and fat) all of which had to be expelled from the body after performing their allotted functions. To this end, enemas were commonly used to force out corrupted food. Enemas were also applied to warriors just before battle on the supposition that this would give them greater strength.

In the lands far to the north, in Central America, which had come to be ruled by the Aztecs from their water-gird city of Tenochtitlán, no less complex was the cause–effect relationship between illness and an afflicted individual. As is now known, the Aztecs had conquered their way to domination only 200 years or so before the arrival of the Spanish.

Guiding them in their endeavors was a pantheon of fierce gods who, each year, demanded their due in human sacrifices. The chosen victims were usually virile young soldiers captured from subordinate peoples. The slaughtered victim's skin was then worn by his captor for some months, as an exercise in humility. The Aztecs believed that only through these blood offerings and ponderings on the transient nature of human life would the coming of the Fifth Sun (the end of the world) be deferred. Integral to these beliefs, they held that happenings in the universe followed an endlessly re-occurring 2,028 year cycle, which was subject to minor re-adjustments at the whim of the gods; hence the need to propitiate them, by sacrifices.

Somewhat paralleling Aztec notions of the macrocosm (the universe, centered on their water-gird capital city) were their notions of the microcosm, individual human beings. Each person's potential fate (when and how he would die, and from what) was related to the precise date in the great year he had been born and its relation to the heavens. However, his own actions in life might alter this fate. This, then, opened the way for the two facets of medicine: the social aspects attended by diviners (the *tlapouhque*), and the physical.

At the physical level, the Aztecs saw the need for the proper flow of bodily juices. They were particularly conscious of the damage which might be done by corrupted water. To counter this threat, their capital city at Tenochtitlán was provided with two aqueducts to bring in fresh, visibly clean water from distant hills. Acutely conscious as well of the damage which might be done by foul smells (analogous to the evil forces of the underworld), the Aztecs bathed themselves frequently (twice-daily, or weekly, depending on their social status) and made much use of cleansing salves and perfumes.

In their concern for public health (clean water) the Aztec, as recent conquerors of central Mexico, were clearly the equal of the ancient Romans, conquerors of western Europe 14 hundred years before. Had Aztec written records survived (rather than being burnt by Spanish Christians), we might possess a New World corpus on the philosophy of medicine equivalent to that which Galen compiled under the stoic, Marcus Aurelius (the emperor who spent most of his adult life on the northern frontier, slaughtering Germans). Yet this was not to be; the Aztec peoples were overtaken by events.

According to a pioneering text in world history revised in 1988, compared to the Spanish, the Aztecs were "technologically primitive." We have seen that this is not at all true. Gross though it is, this example of Eurocentric bias reminds us that, until recently, the writing of history (including medical history) was done almost entirely by scholars who were genetically related to the *victors* of the conflicts of times past. This means that those New World societies that were unfortunate enough to lose wars and to become extinct have nearly always had a bad press.

Further reading

A standard text on the ancient Egyptians is: John F. Nunn, *Ancient Egyptian Medicine* (London: British Museum Press, 1996). See also J. W. Estes, *The Medical Skills of Ancient Egypt* (revised edn Canton, MA, 1993). For specialized articles, see *International Journal of Osteoarchaeology* (from 1990 onward). For New World medicine: Suzanne Alchon, *Native Society and Disease in Colonial Ecuador* (Cambridge University Press, 1991); Brian Fagan, *The Aztecs* (New York: W. H. Freeman, 1984).

Chapter 3

Pluralism in ancient Greece

Introduction

In this chapter I briefly consider elements in the medical and disease history of the societies which constituted classical Greece in the sixth, fifth and fourth centuries BCE (Athens, Sparta, Cos, etc.). I will then quickly touch on the situation in the pagan polities which built directly on ancient Greek legacies. These successor polities were first, the Hellenistic Empire (for our purposes based in Alexandria and Athens) which incorporated the conquests of Alexander the Great (d. 323 BCE) and, second, the Roman Empire, the composite polity surrounding the Mediterranean Sea that was constructed by Augustus Caesar in and after 27 BCE.

To enable us to come to grips with actual (as opposed to fictive) disease and medical reality in the classical world of Greece, it is essential that we realize at the onset that the core set of medical teachings (the "Great Tradition") which came to be known in the West from the eleventh century CE onwards was, in fact, a highly selective distillation of a large body of works written in the fifth and fourth centuries BCE (and later) which came to be known as the Hippocratic Corpus. The word "corpus" however is quite misleading, since it suggests some sort of unity and intellectual coherence.

In reality, as critical twentieth-century scholarship has found, when looked at individually, the authors of the various treatises in this Corpus did not agree among themselves about basic questions such as "What is nature?," "What is the nature of man?," "What is the relationship between man and nature?," "What is disease?," "What is the proper role of a medical specialist?"

In short, when discussing ideas about health and illness in classical Greece, even when dealing with those in the rag-bag of dissonant ideas which is the Hippocratic Corpus, it is essential to think in terms of intellectual diversity. Coming out of this diversity was a considerable degree of medical pluralism among literate practitioners (for example, the practice of "starving a fever" as opposed to "bleeding" a fever victim to rid him of "inappropriate" bodily juices). Even more diverse were the practices (hinted at here and there in the literature) used by run-of-the-mill illiterate curers, and by literate priestly Others.

A second key introductory point which must always be kept in mind is that "formal" medicine in the Classical World was very much the handmaiden of philosophy. In that world (just as in China before 1840 CE) philosophers constituted the intellectual elite. They prided themselves on their ability to use "human reason" to find definitive answers to important questions. Those medical practitioners who actually dealt with patients and tried to make a living in that way were regarded as mere craftsmen. Some few of these medical craftsmen, such as the literate men (women were invisible) who contributed to the Hippocratic Corpus, attempted to improve their own self-image and their status among their fellows by incorporating ideas from one or another of the schools of philosophy into an essay or public disquisition at the forum about what "medicine" (as field) was all about.

Typical of public men in the Ancient World, the claims of these medical craftsmen/writers to expertise and special knowledge were great, but their means of demonstrating the truth of their claims using any tool other than rhetoric were virtually non-existent. Even if one particular orator or essayist happened to hit on what a (Whiggish) modern medical scientist might regard as a credible and accurate medical truth, it would be found that a rival Ancient World orator had used convincing logic to "prove" the opposite. In the absence of modern-style scientific methods to gain practical knowledge of the world around us (unknown before the 1790s CE), there was no way other than the application of verbose prose logic of the sort used to such good effect by the great synthesizer Galen (129 to 200/210 CE) to "prove" that one Ancient World hypothesis about the nature of disease, man, or the cosmos more closely approximated reality than did any rival hypothesis.

At this point some readers may wish to know about the role played by medical personnel who dissected dead bodies or cut up living beings in the interest of learning about human anatomy and the connection between this knowledge and diseases. Unfortunately, surviving evidence is contradictory. Some evidence suggests that in classical times there was some dissection of dead non-human mammals and that in this way it was determined that the brain (an organ ignored by the ancient Egyptians) must have some functions. However, writing a century after Hippocrates, the great categorizer, biologist and philosopher Aristotle – the Schoolmaster of the Western Middle Ages – still held that the heart was the principal vital organ (seat of the soul and passions) and that the brain was merely a sort of regulator and modifier.

Three other points must be mentioned. First, we know that classical Greek notions of the dignity of humankind worked against the dissection of humans, as opposed to animals; unfortunately animal anatomy often was (and is) a misleading guide to human anatomy. Second, we know that in ancient Greece anatomy demonstrations on animals were often given in public and were intended to prove the skills and predictive abilities of one demonstrator as opposed to his rival. These gory shows were not intended to produce new knowledge.

Third, we also know that in late classical times, in Ptolemaic Alexandria the ruler was delighted to serve as Patron of all learning, even if this meant the vivisection of living convicts and slaves drawn from the non-Greek population. Loss of Alexandrian records in the Library fire caused by Julius Caesar (d. 44 BCE) means that we really don't know if the Greek expert, Herophilus (330–260/250 BCE) advanced medical knowledge in any way by carving up living Egyptian males: he seems to have had difficulty in procuring young women for this purpose. In any case we do know that studies of anatomy in eighteenth-century France (scene of the "birth of the clinic") were a dead end when it came to advancing knowledge about infectious diseases and many other sorts of illness. In Hellenistic Greece and Egypt, the relatively new major killer disease was malaria. Understanding of its cause, its course within the body, and how to cure it was not advanced one iota by the study of anatomy.

In Roman times, Galen, the independently wealthy Greek synthesizer of the Hippocratic Corpus who lived near Rome, began his career by working among wounded gladiators in his home town of Pergamon (now in Turkey). Living in the imperial capital at a time when the Roman army was slaughtering its way across the German lands and the Roman populace was satisfying its blood-lust by watching gladiatorial combats in the Colosseum (built soon after 69 CE) Galen would have had abundant opportunities to carry on his studies in human anatomy. However, he may have recognized that this was not a useful way to spend his time since it was at odds with his great project: this was to demonstrate the validity of Humoralism, the retention of a proper balance within the human body by following a *regimen* prescribed by a knowledgeable medical specialist.

Health-seeking pluralism

In 430 BCE, and again in 427, a great pestilence broke out in Athens. At the time that city-state was at the height of its imperial grandeur, the acknowledged leader of much of the Greek world. Its leadership however was being challenged by Sparta and the Peloponnesian League whose invading armies had forced the Athenians on to the defensive behind their Long Walls: there they were pent up in insanitary conditions. In the course of its two outbreaks, the pestilence (we have no way of knowing what it was) killed off a third of the Athenians.

Given that medical doctors found themselves utterly powerless against the "plague" of Athens, their claims to competence in dealing with any illness were thrown further into doubt. Perhaps by coincidence, throughout the Greek world by the last third of the fifth century temples dedicated to the healing god, Asclepius, had became hugely popular. In Rome, symptomatic of growing Greek influence in metaphysical matters, a temple dedicated to the god was established in 291 BCE.

Throughout the Mediterranean world Asclepian temples continued to attract crowds until their functions were taken over by miracle-working Christian saints and shrines in the fourth and fifth centuries CE. Who then was Asclepius?

According to legend, Asclepius was the son of the Greek god Apollo, the same god who had hurtled the darts of killing pestilence against the Greeks around 1200 BCE when they were besieging the city of Troy (as recounted by "Homer" in the *Iliad*). Asclepius' mother however was a mortal woman. Given that Asclepius had this link with humankind, after he had fallen out with Zeus and been killed because he had restored a dead man to life without permission, he was elevated into the ranks of the gods.

The still-extant walls of temples dedicated to Asclepius at Cos, Pergamum, Epidaurus and elsewhere contain plaques commemorating the miraculous cures effected in their precincts. The procedure was for a blind, or crippled, or mentally deranged, or hopelessly afflicted individual to sleep for a night or two in the temple. He or she then dreamed that Asclepius, in one or another of his forms, had appeared and given instructions. The next morning these instructions were interpreted by a priest. According to the commemorative plaques put up by the no longer blind, or the no longer crippled, these instructions had led to a cure. Some of those cured by these miraculous interventions claimed to have been medical practitioners.

In the Greek language, the word "*iatros*" has a variety of meanings. It might mean someone who had persuaded others that he was a medical doctor. At the time there were no teaching hospitals or standard ways of acquiring a medical education. Though some cities at the end of the classical period had taken to appointing a civic physician, the appointment was made after public disquisition between rival contestants. The man who spoke most logically won out, even though his actual ability to effect cures was possibly non-existent. There were no medical licensing institutions or regulatory bodies.

In addition to "medical doctor" the word "*iatros*" can also mean root-cutter, drug-provisioner, midwife, wise woman. People in all of these categories might take upon themselves the role of public curer. In normal circumstances of course, out in the Greek countryside or in the Roman Campagnia, the head of household or his wife served as the first line of defense against illness in the *familia* (the cellular social grouping consisting of the biological family and its slaves). Though specialists admit that they really know very little about the sorts of herbal remedies and drugs used by the common people in classical times, they assume that they were similar to those listed in the books on home remedies published in western Europe from the sixteenth century onwards.

Hints in various places in the literature of ancient Greece suggest that, in addition to herbs and drugs, another locally available avenue of relief from illness lay in the use of incantations. It seems that the *words* of the incantation itself were considered to be efficacious, rather than who said them or the purpose for which they were said. Thus, a head of household might send out a slave to repeat an incantation over a sick horse or a fellow slave in the expectation that it would have the desired effect. In contrast to the situation among the Persians and the Jews, it is thought that the ancient Greeks did not resort to *curses* to cause a disease to attack one of their enemies.

Medicine and the supernatural

Critical research has clearly shown that the supernatural underlay Greek "rationalism" in medicine as in all other fields. Aside from two schools of thought which emerged late in the Hellenistic period, the Methodists and the Empiricists, all other Greek medical writers (including Galen) fully believed that elements of the Divine were to be found everywhere. The sun, the moon, the planets and the stars all contained or reflected aspects of the Divine, as did the everyday world of human experience.

According to the Greeks, and most prominently in the works of Plato (427–*c.* 347 BCE) and his highly erudite and prolific student Aristotle (384–322 BCE), the cosmos and the world of everyday experience could be likened to a ship at anchor in heavy seas. Though the ship veered violently around from one direction to another as it was hit first by one wind and then by another coming in from another side, there was a limit to how far it would move (held fast by its sheet-anchor). Similarly in the cosmos, despite apparent changes, there was underlying stability and order. It was, of course, the duty of the philosopher to discover what this actual reality was (hence Plato's posited World of Perfect Forms).

Now it was, of course, *essential* to the creation of "science" (as we understand it) to hold that there were rules undergirding the workings of the universe. If all humankind had believed that disorder and chaos was what actual reality was all about, not only would the development of "science" have been impossible, so too would the development of ethics and concepts such as virtue, civic duty and restraint. As it was, these concepts – together with the notion of an underlying rule-bound cosmos and world of the everyday – won through to become the dominant element in the Great Tradition. Fittingly enough, Galen (the great medical synthesizer living in the time of the Emperor Marcus Aurelius) wrote an essay entitled, "The best physician is also a philosopher."

Yet, even in the writings of Galen there were three minor mentions of a disturbing concept which had the potential to throw a spanner into the comfortable picture of a rule-governed universe in which a well-endowed person could keep himself in good health by maintaining a proper balance among the "humors" at work within his body. The troublesome concept involved the notion that disease was caused by invisible entities coming in from the outside to attack a person and cause his death. This invisible agency was posited to be an independent force which could strike down anyone whatever his or her status, mode of living or life-style. If the logic of this position were followed through, there would be no need for medical doctors or indeed for any curers. The disease itself would always be master of the situation: Hesiod (in his "Works and Days") had stated as much in the sixth century BCE.

Yet, by the fifth century BCE, this idea (a disease universe of chaos) had been rejected and been replaced by the dictates of philosophy. The self-proclaimed role of the philosopher and the philosopher of medicine was to prove that thinking men who allowed themselves to be governed by sensible rules could *maintain* themselves in good health. The recommended *regimen* was essentially preventive: they were to "do nothing in extreme." Only in this way would their humors be kept in balance.

As goes without saying, humoralism was intensely individualistic. Only a rich man could afford to employ a personal physician who could advise him from day to day on dietary intake, the sexual and exercise requirements appropriate to his temperament and his time of life, and the season of the year, the sign of the zodiac under which he had been born, and the rest.

Philosophical medicine (as synthesized by Galen and later Muslim thinkers) was designed to answer every question. With its multiplicity of answers it could not readily be falsified: in this, doubtless, lay its longevity. It may also be suggested that the doctrine of humoralism provided medical doctors with a distinctive role in society. If, through the accidents of history, they had happened to be deprived of their role as interpreters, they might have permanently disappeared.

Indeed, during the last years of the Roman Empire in the West, hard-faced local secular rulers, most of them recruited from the ranks of provincial armies, decided that Greek-style humoralism and medicine was effete and unmanly, hence unnecessary. By the sixth century CE, except for the tiny Byzantine outpost at Ravenna, the medical profession in the West had ceased to exist.

For the next five hundred years, the future of formal medicine in the Great Tradition lay to the south and east of the Mediterranean, in the world of Islam. To this region we now turn.

Further reading

Leading specialists in the field of Greek medicine include G. E. R. Lloyd; see for example his *Methods and Problems in Greek Science* (Cambridge

University Press, 1990); Vivian Nutton; see for example his "Humoralism" in W. F. Bynum and R. Porter (eds) *Companion Encyclopedia of the History of Medicine* (London: Routledge, 1993) and the late Ludwig Edelstein, *Ancient Medicine* (Baltimore: Johns Hopkins University Press, 1967).

Chapter 4

The evolution of medical systems in the Middle East c. 632 CE to modern times

The Islamic achievement

The Islamic world drew on the medical achievements of the ancient Greco-Roman world and subtly transformed them to fit its own purposes. In this form, they were transmitted to the primitive West and served as the starting point for later Western medicine in the Great Tradition. But equally important in World History, Islamic medicine also built on medical traditions coming from ancient Persian, Arabian and Egyptian sources and created a lasting new synthesis.

The years immediately after the death of the Prophet Muhammad in 632 CE had seen the rapid expansion of Islam beyond the Arabian Peninsula to encompass the whole of the territory of the old Persian Empire in the east, and the Christian provinces of greater Syria and Egypt in the west. To the east, Islam continued its advance and, by the 670s, it had come to incorporate much of what is now Afghanistan and the Indian province known as Sind. Islam's advance also continued in the west, and by 720 it had come to include the whole of North Africa (bringing it to the shores of the Atlantic and the Mediterranean). It had also come to include Sicily and the Iberian Peninsula.

Within two or three generations of their incorporation into the world of Islam, the new provinces sent the most talented of their young men and women to the rapidly growing urban centers of the empire. Beginning first in Baghdad (now in Iraq) until it was wrecked by the Mongols in 1258, and then in Damascus (Syria) and Cairo (Egypt), immigrant and locally born scholars mingled together, exchanging ideas. Coming out of this were new systems of thought about illness that contained elements from several provinces, mixed together in new ways.

As I will explain below, the best known of these systems fed directly into the Great Tradition of Greco–Romano–Arabic medicine which, beginning in the late eleventh century, was introduced into the West (this learned tradition would form the basis of the medical curriculum in Western universities until the eighteenth century). Another of the systems of the Middle

East (synthesized in and before the early fourteenth century) came to be called the "Medicine of the Prophet." Today (in its Islamic form rather than in its popular variant) the "Medicine of the Prophet" continues strong among Muslim immigrant populations in the West.

In the early Islamic centuries, the technological innovation that greatly assisted in building up new syntheses in medicine, natural philosophy, theology and in other areas of scholarly concern was the making of paper. Brought in from China, by 750 paper was being produced in all the great cities of the Islamic world. Books made up of sheets of paper bound together around a single spine were much more convenient to use, to carry around, and to store in great libraries, than were old-fashioned scrolls made of sheep-skin or papyri.

They were, of course, produced by hand. A master would slowly read out a scholarly work and scribes would copy down what he said. Depending on how many scribes he employed, ten or fifteen or more copies of a 300-page book could be produced in a few weeks. It was in this way that, by 1236, (when it was burnt by crusading Christians) the great Library in Islamic Cordoba (in Andalusia, Spain) had built up a collection said to number 400,000 books.

Islamic medicine: Classical Period

It is now generally accepted that, by the early tenth century, leading Islamic physicians had gone far beyond the ancient Greeks in the study and practice of medicine. One of the greatest of their number was undoubtedly Abu Bakr Muhammad al-Razi (865–925 CE). Born in the city of Rayy in northern Persia during the period of weakening Abbasid rule, al-Razi spent part of his adult career in Baghdad (the Caliph's seat of government) and the remainder in Rayy (where he was on good terms with the local governor). In both cities he served as director of a local hospital.

In his studies al-Razi was able to bring together what he regarded as the best of the traditions of the ancient world: Greek, Syriac, Persian, with a bit of ancient Egyptian thrown in. But unlike most of his predecessors, al-Razi did not allow himself to be overwhelmed by the grandeur of the book-learning of the past. Instead, in his day-to-day interaction with patients, he made it a practice to note down the specifics of each case and to draw up conclusions which very often were at odds with the conclusions of earlier masters.

Several of the clinical observations al-Razi made in Baghdad have been translated into Western languages. These show that his patients came from the neighborhood around the Muqtadiri Hospital where he taught. They included door-keepers and craftsmen and their wives and other quite ordinary people. The diseases and conditions al-Razi dealt with included perforated kidneys (leading to symptoms of fever), diarrheal diseases, inflammation of a man's sexual organs, a woman's miscarriage, and eye diseases. In the case of al-Husain Ibn ʿAbdawaih's daughter, al-Razi found that she was suffering from a mild case of smallpox and, through appropriate treatment (doubtless much aided by the healing processes of nature), he was able to save her eyesight.

In his clinical practice, al-Razi had several assistants who seem to have dealt with routine cases. Yet he kept himself immensely busy with seeing patients, with reading and discussing ancient texts with students, and with writing, writing, writing. Specialists tell us that al-Razi wrote a total of 61 medical treatises. Of these, only 32 are still preserved in one or another of the world's archives and only nine have been translated from the Arabic into a western European language. In other words, much of what al-Razi wrote has been lost or has not been critically studied in the West. As a result, while awaiting translations from Arabic, current English-language assessments of his achievements can only be provisional.

The Greek legacy underlying al-Razi's work: Galen and Hippocrates

The most recent of the Greeks on whose works al-Razi drew was the great synthesizer, Galen (129–200/210 CE) who lived near Rome in the time of the Emperor Marcus Aurelius. We now know that Galen had been extremely selective in his choice of the Hippocratic works and other ancient Greek sources from which he chose to quote.

At its full-blown best in the fifth and fourth centuries BCE, as we saw in Chapter 3, ancient Greek medicine had accepted the importance of *open* intellectual inquiry and of medical pluralism. It had not cared that some groups of medical writers utterly contradicted other writers. Galen on the other hand, coming much later as synthesizer and simplifier, had picked up only certain threads from the ancient Greek medical past, and by so doing he had all but closed the door of intellectual inquiry. Only in our own time – when in practical terms Hippocrates, the other ancient Greeks, and Galen have all become irrelevant to actual medical research – have historians of medicine finally discovered how instrumental Galen was in skewing the long-term development of the medical profession.

Galen, as systemizer and simplifier had worked within a complex paradigm that posited a balanced constitution as equivalent to good health, and an unbalanced constitution as equivalent to some sort of disease condition. Galen was also very much aware of the need to keep the medical profession in being by providing it with fee-paying patrons/clients. Accordingly, he had argued that each individual client had his/her own particular balance: this balance gradually changed as the client progressed from childhood to youth to adulthood and on to old-age. Within this schema, the role of a physician was to understand the particular characteristics of his client and (for a fee) to prescribe a proper *regimen* for him to follow. Improper foods and excessive eating were obviously to be warned against, as were insufficient exercise or too much exercise of the wrong sort. According to Galen, moderation in all things and a worry-free existence was the key to health.

Yet, going far beyond what an intelligent layman might have been able to figure out for himself (without the expense of paying a consultant physician) Galen's paradigm also posited the division of the theory of medicine into three parts. These were the theory of the "natural" causes of disease as a deviation from the normal, the theory of "causes" and the theory of "signs."

There were seven "natural" things: the four elements (earth, air, fire, water): complexions (nine in number, a combination of hot and cold, wet and dry); the four humors (phlegm, yellow bile, black bile and blood); the four members (the brain, the heart, the liver, the testicles – two in number but counted as one); the three forces; the two actions (i.e. unconscious digestive processes and conscious movement); the three spirits; the three types of sickness. In addition, there were the six "non-naturals." The first five, according to Galen, were climate, motion and rest, diet, sleeping patterns, evacuation and sexuality; the sixth consisted of afflictions of the soul. Even a quick scan of this listing of categories of things and forces (each of which had a complex meaning) will convince the reader that for Galen and his followers "medicine" was really a branch of philosophy: only a well-educated specialist could begin to understand it.

Abu Bakr al-Razi, while in Baghdad and later in Rayy, attempted to get a grip on these Galenic notions. But as an inquiring scholar, he also attempted to come to terms with what "Hippocrates" himself had said, uncorrupted by Galen. A body of writings attributed to "Hippocrates" (a man or group of men who had lived on the Mediterranean island of Cos c. 460 to 377 BCE) had been collected and collated at the great library complex at Alexandria around 250 BCE, during the Ptolemaic era of Egyptian history.

Among the Hippocratic writings that came into the hands of al-Razi by way of the Alexandria Library and successor collections further east were medical texts such as "Epidemics" and "Airs, Waters, Places." The latter attributed disease outbreaks to the special characteristics of a particular place. "Airs, Waters, Places" also suggested that people living in hot climes would have different physiological characteristics from people living in a cold mountainous zone or from people (like the inhabitants of the Greek island of Cos) who lived in a nicely balanced temperate zone.

The triumph of scholastic philosophy over medicine

In the course of his career (continuing until 925), al-Razi brought down upon himself the hatred of three categories of people. First, as a learned man who subjected some elements of the received medical wisdom of the past to the test of empirical observation, he was seen as trespassing into the domain occupied by empirics. Empirics were seen to be uneducated (in the formal sense of the word) illiterate people who claimed to be able to cure diseases, for a fee (in the West, empirics continued to be the bane of professionally educated medical doctors until the early twentieth century when they were subsumed into one or other of the schools of "alternative medicine").

The Middle Eastern empirics living in al-Razi's time who kept at their trade for several years were likely to have found that curative substance "x" was more effective than substance "y" in correcting a particular disease condition. However, as al-Razi and other learned men kept pointing out, empirics (by definition) had no theoretical understanding of why substance "x" worked and substance "y" did not. It was this lack of theoretical understanding which caused them to be regarded as profit-seeking opportunists whom educated medical doctors should crush.

But, in retrospect, more damaging for the cause of actual progress in medical knowledge was the fact that empirics lacked an institutional way to transmit their knowledge from one generation to the next. The insights some few of them might have arrived at were very rarely handed on to anyone else. Given the importance of trade secrets, and the distrust with which a master regarded his apprentices, when a tight-lipped empiric died, his insights died with him.

More damaging to al-Razi than his professed contempt for illiterate empirics (generally people without much political clout) was the contempt with which he himself was regarded by the teachers of the Law, the jurists and the theologians. In the Islamic world in the tenth century, with the increasing fragmentation of political authority and the establishment of independent principalities on the fringes of empire, jurists centered in Baghdad were growing increasingly bold in insisting that they alone had the competence to trace the roots of all knowledge back to Allah, either as it was written down in the Holy Qur'an or as found in one of the many sayings of the Prophet, the *hadith*.

It was jurists and theologians largely resident in Baghdad who decided which *hadith* were authentic and which were not. Initially, they turned their systemizing minds to the Law. Though seen earlier as issuing forth from the sayings of the Prophet Muhammad, subject to some degree of personal interpretation, the Law (now rigorously interpreted by Baghdad-based jurists) came to be regarded as formal and fixed, no longer subject to personal judgement. In their hands, the Law was now said to represent the consensus of the community against which individual protest was futile.

Having all but closed the door to individual reasoning in the field of the Law, Baghdad-based jurists and their close allies, the theologians and the philosophers, turned their attention to medicine. In an attempt to counter their usurpation of interpretive authority here, al-Razi (as secular doctor and as a Muslim) pointed out that very little about sickness or curing was mentioned in the Qur'an. One of the three small notices found there said that Muslims should not personally hold cripples, the blind or the sick in contempt. The Qur'an also advised that honey might have curative power, and that believers should wash before settling down to prayer. Quite unlike the Christian Bible (which incidentally was not translated into Arabic until long after the Qur'an had achieved its final form), the Holy Book of Islam said nothing else on the subject of medicine on which theologians could build.

Al-Razi, in an attempt to maintain the independence of medicine as an essentially secular field as it had been under the ancient Greeks, also pointed out that Allah had given humankind the use of Reason. From this it followed that Reason participated in the Divine Substance. Al-Razi also pointed out that the Prophet Muhammad had stressed that, before Allah, all believers were equal. Al-Razi glossed this to read that all educated men were entitled to interpret God's word to the best of their own understanding. Yet al-Razi, as medical scholar, was no match for the combined weight of the Baghdad jurists and theologians who claimed that they alone had the prerogative of selecting and remembering *hadith*. Some of these newly remembered *hadith* proved that medicine (like all other learned fields) fell under the purview of specialist scholars in religion.

At the same time that he was being grounded by the theologians, al-Razi was also being attacked by philosophers. In theory, philosophers concerned themselves with secular matters, as defined by their scholarly brothers in theology who, in theory, specialized in the study of the laws of God.

Even as al-Razi was at work observing the symptoms of his patients and writing up his critical observations, Islamic philosophers were assigning themselves the task of "reconciling" secular written learning preserved from ancient Greece with Divine Revelation. The tool the philosophers used was logic, as defined by Aristotle (384–322 BCE) sometime advisor to the quint-essential authoritarian, Alexander the Great.

We now know that in the world of pre-modern science and pre-modern medicine, almost any preconceived idea (no matter how weird) could be demonstrated to be "true" by the manipulation of complex logical forms (such as analogies and correspondences). Indeed, for the medieval followers of Aristotle, the philosophic beauty of any medical concept lay in its sym-metry, its correspondence with other aspects of nature, and with other philo-sophic ideals. For such men of medicine, the working out of Aristotle's philosophic "logic" became an end in itself.

Ibn Sina

This was certainly the case with the principal personage with whom (outside the Islamic heartlands) the future of Middle-Eastern (and Western) formal medicine lay, Ibn Sina (980–1037 CE). In the West, Ibn Sina was known as Avicenna.

In a way not uncommon among members of a profession which is not sure of its direction, Ibn Sina held al-Razi's memory in contempt, and famously said that al-Razi should have contented himself with playing about with urine and excrement, and left the practice of "proper" medicine to others. But in describing his own education, Ibn Sina stated that he had been trained in metaphysics, mathematics, the rational sciences, logic, in the Qur'an, and in the sciences of the Arabic language: he made no mention of having received any formal instruction in medicine. This, however, did not prevent him from writing, rather extensively, about the subject.

Ibn Sina compiled a book, simply known as the *Canon* (the *Kitab al-Qanum*) which in an estimated one million words claimed to contain the whole of the medical wisdom of the Ancient World. In fact it is only a carefully selected fragment of that wisdom: it omitted mention of great chunks of the medical past which were at odds with Ibn Sina's basic interpretation. Yet fragmentary though it was, the *Canon* was the agency through which the Greek inheritance, and Galen's interpretation of that inheritance, was transferred to the West.

Following the rules of Aristotelian logic, the *Canon* is organized into books, chapters, sub-chapters, headings and sub-headings. It has all the advantages of a book for teenage students which can be easily memorized even though students don't know what key words mean. It was this scholastic triumph of rote learning over medicine that was the principal contribution which, in due course, the Islamic world passed on to the West. Initially, this was done through translations of the *Canon* from Arabic into Latin by Constantinus Africanus. Constantinus was a Christian monk from Tunis – hence his knowledge of Arabic – who lived between *c.* 1020 and 1087. For many years he worked at Monte Casino, north of Naples. We will mention him again in Chapter 8 when we further pursue the link between Islamic medicine (as transmitter of the Great Tradition) and the medieval and early modern West.

In addition to its vitally important role in the making of the West, the *Canon* also had a great future ahead of it far to the east. While Ibn Sina was still at work, Mahmud of Ghazni led Islamic armies into the Punjab and beyond, defeated local Hindu forces (1001–25), and placed the newly acquired lands under the nominal authority of the Abbasid caliph. Because of the coincidence of timing and the role of newly synthesized ideas in conquered provinces (easier to communicate than were the complexities found in original sources) Ibn Sina's *Canon* came to form the basis of *Unani Tibb* medicine in India (see Chapter 5).

Specialists in the history of Islamic medicine have reminded us of an important point. This is that in the case of simple peoples (eleventh-century Seljuk Turks, or Punjabi, or Europeans) who were acquiring foreign ideas through a crash-course method, the impact made by multiple copies of a book of synthesis tended to be more profound than that made by a single copy of an earlier book that (seen from the modern scholarly perspective) was more intellectually stimulating.

This was certainly the case with Ibn Sina's *Canon* when contrasted with the writings of al-Razi (with whom the future did *not* lie). In libraries in Istanbul (the capital of the Ottoman Turks and, after the Ottoman conquest of Cairo in 1517, the chief city of the Islamic world), at least 60 rather tatty copies of Ibn Sina's *Canon* are currently found, compared to only one or two bits of al-Razi's work. The fine state of preservation of the latter (compared to the works of Ibn Sina) suggests that al-Razi was seldom consulted. In Turkish-ruled lands (as in the West), the medical future belonged to Ibn Sina.

The role of formal medicine in Islamic heartlands after 1050

Important insights into the role played by formal medicine and medical doctors in the Islamic heartlands a century and a quarter after the death of al-Razi (925 CE) are provided by the medical writer and practitioner, ʿAli ibn Ridwan (998–1068). Ibn Ridwan lived in Fustat, adjacent to Cairo.

In Ibn Ridwan's time, Egypt was an independent province, having been conquered in 962 by a Shi'ite group from Morocco, the Fatimids. They would continue to rule Egypt until 1171 when they were ousted by the great Sunni general known in the West as Saladin. Under the Fatimids, Cairo became a central emporium in the trade in spices, drugs and fine luxury products with India, and beyond India, the trade with China.

With our modern knowledge about the spread of contagious diseases coming in from other places in the bodies of infected people, or on trade goods, or in fleas on rats, we recognize that Cairo during Ibn Ridwan's time was in a particularly vulnerable position. Though none of the most serious disease killers (such as bubonic plague) were endemic in Egypt, Cairo did lie at the crossing-point of two major trading routes, each of which could be easily traversed by killer disease agents.

One route lay with the boat traffic on the Nile, going north to the port cities of Alexandria and Rossetta, and south to Nubia (with its gold mines) and on to sub-Saharan Africa (with its ivory and slaves). Another trading route connected Cairo with India, going south down the Nile to the city of Qus, then overland to the Red Sea and onwards to India. Cairo was also a major refurbishing point for Muslim pilgrims traveling on their Haj to Mecca and Medina, the Holy Cities in the Arabian peninsula. In short, it was at the center of transport networks which were liable to bring in all sorts of dread diseases.

In his treatise "On the prevention of bodily ills in Egypt," Ibn Ridwan reminds us of the inability of medical doctors to control major disease disasters. Writing in the 1050s, he said that in the previous twenty years Egypt had witnessed five epidemics, though only one of them had been cata-strophic. We know from other sources that just after Ibn Ridwan laid down his pen, Egypt suffered from a particularly serious famine which lasted from 1065 to 1072. With it came a host of famine-related diseases.

This late eleventh-century famine was caused by successive failures of the River Nile to rise to its normal height during the season of inundations. Because there was virtually no rainfall in Egypt, in ordinary years the water needed to nurture the crops was trapped during the inundation behind specially constructed mud dams. But when the Nile failed for several suc-cessive years to rise to its usual height, food reserves would be used up and people starved to death. In the terrible late 1060s and early 1070s, surviv-ing people were forced to eat roots and dogs, cats and other small living things. Putrid water supplies led to many diarrheal diseases. Infant mortal-ity rates may well have reached 500 per 1,000 live births a year. This was greatly in excess of the normal rate which was probably around 200 per 1,000.

Ibn Ridwan was well aware of the consequences of epidemics but, as a medical doctor, it was up to him to try to explain their causes. In his "On the prevention of bodily ills in Egypt," (written in the 1050s) he fell back on the explanatory words of the Ancients found in the Hippocratic Corpus. Thus, in his chapter "On the causes of pestilence," he stated that epidemics were caused by four categories of causes: "a change in the quality of the air, a change in the quality of the water, a change in the quality of the food, and a change in the quality of psychic events." This stress on "change" as causal agent went back to the Hippocratic idea that the natives of a particular place had become fully acclimatized to its peculiarities and had evolved an appropriate life-style (*regimen*). Any major "change" in their homeland environment would bring about disease.

For Ibn Ridwan, writing in the 1050s, "change in the air" meant an unusual change, not a standard seasonal change. The air would suddenly become abnormally wetter or dryer, hotter or colder, or it might become mixed with a "corruption" (i.e. a stench arising from decaying organic matter or corpses on a battlefield) brought in from a distant place, say the "Sudan" or "Ethiopia" (general terms, not specific places), which had then descended on Egypt, causing an epidemic.

Still on the topic of "air," Ibn Ridwan suggested that if large numbers of people in Egypt began to worry because of a sharp rise in food prices, and forgot to follow their customary *regimen* and to wash themselves, their bodies would begin to stink, leading to a putrification rising into the atmos-phere, then descending on Cairo, causing an epidemic. Ibn Ridwan went on to say that the intensity of any particular epidemic depended on the nature of its originating causes. If two or more causes combined (war in the "Sudan" – leaving many rotting corpses – and famine in Egypt) the illness would be swifter in its killing, and more intense, than would other-wise be the case.

In all these conclusions, Ibn Ridwan presented an explanation of epidemic disease causation which (for his contemporaries) was both intellectually satisfying (it had answers for everything) while, at the same time, intellectually respectable (it was based on the wisdom of ancient authority). Moreover, though Ibn Ridwan (an Egyptian Muslim) may not have been aware of it, his explanatory system had genuinely Egyptian roots. In pharaonic times, the Egyptians had credited many otherwise unexplained disease conditions to the foul fumes arising from putrifying organic matter. By using this causal explanation, beloved of the Ancients, Ibn Ridwan, writing in the 1050s CE made it clear that there was nothing medical doctors (such as himself) could be expected to do to prevent or to control an epidemic.

In addition to his treatise "On the prevention of bodily ills in Egypt," Ibn Ridwan is interesting in other ways. Let us turn to the manner in which he and others like him were trained in the mysteries of medicine.

Medical education and hospitals

Because Ibn Ridwan's parents were not wealthy, he had to support himself after he reached puberty and decided to take up the practice of medicine. So he dabbled in astrology. Then as now astrology worked on the premise that the creator God had placed humankind at the center of the universe, and that the movement of the stars and other planets was directly related to the activities of each earth-bound human.

With the money he earned from astrology, Ibn Ridwan purchased books containing the ancient wisdom of Galen and Hippocrates and disciplined himself to understand the deeper meanings of what he read. Though he was largely self-taught, on occasion, to ensure that he had not drifted entirely off course, he attended lessons given by a senior medical doctor.

At these sessions (which were a standard part of all formal medical training) students read aloud from one of the Masters. Competent teachers habitually stopped students who had mis-read or mis-interpreted a sentence. However senior physician-teachers whose only interest was to collect the fees the students paid them would allow students to forge ahead, uncorrected.

After a full-time student had been at his books for several years, a senior physician might suggest that he take up the practice of medicine. At the time, none of the great cities of the Islamic world boasted of a central medical testing service. What often happened instead was that a young man's patron (not necessarily a doctor) brought his name to the attention of the local market inspector. This police agent then would give the young man permission to practice medicine.

In long-established Islamic cities, such as Baghdad in the time of al-Razi (late ninth century) or Cairo in the time of Saladin (after 1171), aspiring doctors sometimes trained at medical hospitals. These hospitals were founded by rich donors as acts of piety (charity being one of the central tenets of

Islam). The terms of the establishment would be written up in a *Waqf* document which would be deposited in the local hall of records. The document would stipulate which pieces of landed property would pay in rent, in perpetuity, for the maintenance of the hospital. Status considerations among donors, mixed with Islamic religious tenets, meant that many of these hospitals were fine, two- or three-story, stone-built buildings, with impressive large rooms and courtyards. We should remind ourselves that in earlier times, in the world of ancient Greece and Rome, there had been no such thing as hospitals for ordinary people.

In the urban Islamic world, it seems that only famous medical doctors were invited to practice in hospitals. Arriving in the wards before dawn and staying until noon, they attended to the medical needs of these who formed the hospital's principal clientele – the poor and the hopelessly disabled. Some medical doctors specialized in repairing broken arms and legs. However, a physician who used treatments such as an amputation which led to death from gangrene would soon lose the respect of his potential clientele. Accordingly, most hospital doctors did not use invasive techniques.

In the Islamic world, there was considerable disincentive to learn about human anatomy at first hand by cutting up the bodies of the dead. Works of Galen, copied and re-copied over the centuries, contained several sketches of anatomical parts, based (it is said) on drawings of the inner workings of monkeys, cats and dogs. In the absence of inquiring minds, these drawings of non-human animal parts were seen as satisfactory.

In any case, according to the Qur'an, the human dead would all rise when the Archangel Gabriel sounded the final trumpet and they were summoned to be judged. At that time it would not be proper if they were missing body parts (other than the foreskin of the penis, all Muslim males having been circumcised before they reached puberty). Moreover, many Muslims thought that the dead would still feel pain if their corpses were hacked about. In a properly ordered world, a dead Muslim was buried (with all her or his body parts complete) within 24 hours of death.

Within a hospital, treatment was free, as befitted a charitable institution. One can however assume that, much like the situation in the West until early in the twentieth century, most people who entered a hospital expected to die there. But at least in cities in the Islamic heartland, they could expect to die in pleasant surroundings. There were an abundance of trees and fountains in the courtyard at the center of the stone-built building. Within, there were well ventilated separate wards for men and for women.

By conducting their early morning practice in a hospital, medical doctors demonstrated that they were charitably inclined, and willing to sacrifice their time to the common good. In the afternoon, back in their private offices, they attended to the needs of fee-paying clients.

Less famous doctors, not found in hospitals, tended to team up in pairs and to practice in offices located near the city market. Organized in this way, one or other of the doctors was likely to be on hand when a request came in for emergency service. Existing records from old city Cairo from the eleventh and twelfth centuries suggest that doctors were quite willing to ride far out into the countryside to attend to the medical needs of the fee-paying rural sick. From small fragments of written evidence, we are led to assume that in most provincial cities and in some of the larger villages, there were one or two medical doctors on hand to serve the needs of the public.

In Egypt under the ʿabbasids, beginning from the time of Saladin (1171–93), Sunni Islam insisted that all "people of the book" should be allowed to practice medicine. This meant that many of the medical doctors for whom records survive were Jews. Coptic Christians also served as doctors, as of course did Muslims. As bearers of ancient wisdom, dating back to Galen and Hippocrates, the social standing of a doctor whatever his confessional preference, largely depended on his reputation for deep learning in ancient wisdom. Well-read, well-bred medical doctors who carried themselves like gentlemen were frequently employed at the court of a Sultan or Caliph or military commander. While at Court medical doctors doubtless spent much of their time giving their patron advice on the *regimen* he should follow in order to preserve good health. They knew that prevention was far easier than cure. However, medically approved cures did exist.

Drugs

As we know from the writing of Ibn Ridwan of Cairo (eleventh century) Egypt's trade with India brought in an increasingly rich cornucopia of exotic new drugs. The 300 or so medicines used in the ninth century had, by his time, expanded in number to nearly 3,000. One of the skills required of a physician was to write up a proper prescription. Contemporary theory held that the greater the number of the drugs it contained, the more effective the medicine would be, of course taking into account the particular characteristics and "complexion" of the patient.

We know from existing eleventh- and twelfth-century Cairene records that drug dealers (pharmacists) were a distinct professional group. However, we also know that a proper physician generally took it upon himself to mix the drugs needed by his fee-paying patients. Inventories of doctors' offices list their standard equipment – scales, measuring spoons, bottles and containers of various shapes and sizes. Seeing all this equipment in their doctor's office assured a patient that the practitioner was a proper doctor rather than a mere charlatan. Indeed, as doctors knew very well, in the final analysis, confidence in the abilities of one doctor and lack of confidence in another made all the difference in deciding which of them to turn to. However, there were other alternatives. To these we now turn.

Forms of the Prophet's medicine: the popular and the elite

One of these alternatives was what, among the unlettered populace, was called "the medicine of the Prophet." This was a loose, somewhat incoherent collection of ideas about health, disease and medicine that was found in one or another of the Middle Eastern regions in the centuries just after it had been brought within the World of Islam, for example, in the mid-seventh, eight and ninth centuries in upper Egypt (bordering Nubia) or in eastern Persia. I will say more about this cluster of medical forms in a moment. But first it is useful just to mention the existence of the second alternative, confusingly also termed the "medicine of the Prophet." Here, the term refers to the formalized, intellectually coherent systems created by members of the learned elite sometime after the year 1100.

We turn now to the popular level, "medicine of the Prophet," as understood by the ordinary people in the street. As we have already seen, the Prophet Muhammad (d. 632) began life as a merchant in Mecca, a principal trading center in the interior of the Arabian peninsula. We have also seen that medical theory did not figure prominently in the revelations he had from Allah which he insisted should sweep away the polytheistic ideas and practices known before then in Mecca and elsewhere in Arabia.

Yet, within the Qur'an (the written record of these revelations), it was stated that Allah saw to it that there was a cure for each of the disease conditions he had inflicted on humankind – excepting only old age. The Qur'an also made it crystal clear that Allah's power was unlimited. This did not rule out the existence of malevolent, small-scale supernatural beings – *jinn* (plural, the singular is *jinni*) – who could be causal agents of disease and death.

The incorporation of *jinn* into Muhammad's explanatory system permitted the survival of a host of pre-existing popular ideas about the problems posed by ill-health and disease. In Egypt, for example, the "Prophet's medicine" included folk ideas dating back to the Old, Middle and New Kingdoms and re-interpreted in succeeding periods – the Persian, Ptolemaic and Romano-Coptic. Nile Valley dwellers also absorbed disease causal ideas from their nomadic neighbors in the deserts, the Bedouin.

One folk idea common to Egypt and the rest of the early Islamic world held that diseases were sent in from the outside through the agency of a *jinni*. This threat could be warded off by the wearing of special amulets.

And given the standard Islamic teaching that it was "natural" and normal for young adult women to be healthy and to bear children, in Egypt another folk idea held that women whose marriages were barren were obviously suffering from a mystic disease. This could be countered by engaging in a special ritual. For example, on three successive Fridays (in Islam, Friday is the holy day of the week), during the time of the principal noon-day prayer at the village mosque, barren women walked seven times counter-clockwise around the exterior walls of a Coptic church. As institution, the Coptic Church had long pre-dated the coming of Islam; its buildings were seen to represent mystic power because they were very old.

Medicine of the Prophet for elites

It will be noticed that the popular-level "Prophet's medicine" I have just discussed had not as yet differentiated itself from ancient Greek medical ideas. However, a few years after the death of al-Razi (925), and particularly after the years 1095 to 1106, learned Muslims became increasingly conscious of the need to do so.

Coming out of all this, was the formalization of the "medicine of the Prophet" for the elite, eventually represented in near final form by Ibn Qayyim al-Jawziyya's fourteenth-century treatise of that name. Born in Damascus in 1262, the author died in 1350 at the ripe old age of 88. It is important to notice that Ibn Qayyim was a jurist (learned in the law). He had no special training in medicine. Indeed in his hierarchy of values, the discipline of medicine was clearly subordinate to the higher discipline, the study of God's law.

In his treatise, the Syrian jurist confronted Greco-Roman "scientific" medicine head on. He clearly stated that there were two categories of disease. Diseases "of the heart" (by which he meant "diseases of the soul") could only be prevented by coming to a better knowledge of, and fully accepting, the laws and ways of God. Indeed, for all the diseases caused by stubborn unwillingness fully to accept God's laws ("sickness of heart," heartache, melancholia, suicidal despair) Ibn Sina's eleventh-century compendia of Greco-Roman medicine was (according to Ibn Qayyim) utterly useless.

Yet, in his mind-over-body approach, Ibn Qayyim fully accepted that there were a wide range of diseases which were strictly physical in origin. Some of these could be cured simply by resort to its opposite. For example, hunger as malaise could be corrected by eating: for these conditions no medical advice was necessary. However, there remained other conditions for which specialized knowledge was required: for these a good Muslim should resort to a physician. Indeed, to pound this point home, Ibn Qayyim quoted a *hadith* in which the Prophet, when queried by a sick disciple about what he should do, ordered the disciple to take himself off immediately to a qualified medical doctor. For diseases of this sort, the Prophet did not feel obliged to effect a miracle cure, or suggest that his followers in the centuries to come should validate their faith by performing miracles.

Another central point which emerges from Ibn Qayyim's use of this particular *hadith* (ordering a believer to seek a physician) was that Muslims were not expected to be fatalists, blindly accepting all disease as something sent down from Allah, against which human intervention was futile. The mis-interpretation of Islam, as the religion of fatalists when confronted by disease, dates from the late seventeenth century onwards when agents of the West in the Middle East and India came to feel that they alone were progressive and "scientific." Part of the mirror image of this conceit was that all Muslims were fatalists.

Among Westerners, Ibn Qayyim's "medicine of the Prophet" was all but forgotten, probably because it did not fit into their stereotype of what a Muslim was. The first English translation was only published in 1998. Yet, among the several million Muslims living in the West, possession of at least parts of Ibn Qayyim's Arabic-language text has long been seen as a necessary hallmark of continued Islamic identity.

Popular medical practices

Before the coming of what the cosmopolitan urban elite regard as "Modern times" (with the Germ Theory, penicillin and injections), the Islamic Middle East could be characterized by its acceptance of medical pluralism: if it works, use it. Among other things, medical pluralism included resort to the tombs of holy saints.

These dead men or women were thought to intercede with God in time of illness or distress. In medieval Cairo, one of the most famous of these holy shrines was that of the woman saint Sayyidah Zaynab. In strict theory Sunni Islam did not recognize saints (seen as a primitive Christian invention). Resort to healing saints was thus not sanctioned by the teachers of the Law and Theology at Cairo's great Islamic university, Al Azhar, founded in 962. However, teachers from Al Azhar were generally in attendance (as indeed they still are) near the courtyard of the mosque and shrine of Sayyidah Zaynab where women gathered just before they entered the tomb chamber of the healing saint.

Two kilometers further to the south, Cairene Christians joined with Muslims (as they still do) in prayers of supplication at the domed tomb shrine of Imam al-Shafi. This then was another application of the aphorism al-Razi (of Rayy and Baghdad) often mentioned in his writings.

For al-Razi the triangle of healing consisted of the sick one, the sickness and the doctor. In the popular understanding, in certain instances, the "doctor" was the healing saint, the sickness was the effect of a disease entity, and the sick one was a person who had faith in the capacity of the saint to effect a cure, or at least to resolve her or his immediate distress. For these people medicine was holistic. They understood that the burden of disease could only be eased by the grit and strong-willed determination of the sick one and her/his loved ones. In this lay the wisdom of the ages.

Further reading

There are only a few up-to-date studies on Islamic medicine. In English, the best are by Lawrence Conrad and Michael Dols. Lawrence Conrad, "Arab-Islamic Medicine," in W. F. Bynum and Roy Porter (eds) *Companion Encyclopedia of the History of Medicine* (London: Routledge, 1993), 676–727; Lawrence Conrad, "Epidemic Disease in Formal and Popular Thought in Early Islamic Society," in Terence Ranger and Paul Slack (eds) *Epidemics and Ideas: essays on the historical perception of pestilence* (Cambridge: Cambridge University Press, 1992), 77–99; Michael Dols, *Medieval Islamic Medicine: Ibn Ridwan's treatise "on the prevention of bodily ills in Egypt"* (Berkeley: University of California Press, 1984); Michael Dols, *The Black Death in the Middle East* (Princeton, NJ: Princeton University Press, 1977). An excellent introduction to transculturalism, in French, is Danielle Jacquart and Françoise Micheau, *La Médecine Arabe et l'Occident Médiéval* (Paris: Editions Maisonneuve et Larose, 1996). For sample texts see: Max Meyerhof, "Thirty-Three Clinical Observations by Rhazes (*c.* 900 AD)," in Penelope Johnstone (ed.) *Studies in Medieval Arabic Medicine: theory and practice* (London: Variorum Reprints, 1984), 321–56. For the Prophet's medicine, see Penelope Johnstone's translation in the Islamic Texts Society, *Medicine of the Prophet* (1998).

Chapter 5

Health and disease on the Indian subcontinent before 1869

Harappan civilization: a false start?

Archaeological excavations carried out in the late 1850s began to uncover, much to everyone's surprise, the extensive remains of a very ancient civilization along the Indus River and its tributaries in what is now northwest India and Pakistan. Before the dig began no one had had any idea that this particular civilization had ever existed.

Dating back to the time of the Old Kingdom in Egypt (around 3000 BCE), this long-lost cultural grouping (the "Harappan civilization") was centered on two large stone-built cities (Harappa and Mohenjo-Daro), each with 20 or 30,000 inhabitants. In addition to its very sizeable urban populations living behind massive defensive walls which in some places were 13 feet thick and 13 feet high, the Harappan civilization also included scores of large dependent villages.

With its tens of thousands of people, this riverine civilization lasted for an estimated 1,300 years. Then, around 1700 BCE it disappeared beneath the mud and sands heaped up by the Indus and its tributaries, perhaps in the course of a series of severe seasonal monsoons. In the wake of these ecological disasters (or perhaps just before they occurred, a possibility hinted at below), the Harappan ruling elite completely disappeared. They took with them all memory of the great civilization they had earlier created.

However, it is likely that several thousand ordinary, once urban-dependent Harappan people continued to live not too far away in the same disease zone in what were now degraded farming communities. Over time, these ordinary peoples' descendants did not find it necessary to "remember" through the media of oral history (see Chapter 1) that their ancestors had once been slaves or menials under a governing elite who had lived in congested great cities.

In its prime, the urban-based Harappan civilization almost certainly contained enough people to maintain several "crowd diseases" (among them, measles, malaria and smallpox). As suggested earlier, for any of these diseases to come into existence (through species jumping and natural selection) it was necessary for sizeable human populations to live in close proximity to

domesticated cattle. In Harappan communities this criteria was met: archae-
ological discoveries include numerous images of bulls. These creatures
required mates. Almost certainly, cattle herding was one of the mainstays
of Harappan civilization.

By way of contrast, as we saw in Chapter 2, in the hinterlands of the
large urban centers in Central and South America, before the coming of
the Europeans in 1492, there was a complete absence of wild cattle and
horses, and of pigs and camels and other mammals (other than dogs) that
could be domesticated and made to live in close contact with humankind.
Going along with this, there were no mass killer infectious diseases in urban
pre-Columbian America.

Harappan governing elites saw to it that their cities were provided with
supplies of clean running water and with sewer systems. Going beyond this
elementary sanitary precaution, on better quality streets in Mohenjo-Daro
and Harappa, most houses had separate little rooms for toilets. The waste
products went into the city sewer system rather than into ordinary people's
drinking water supplies (as sometimes happened much later in early
Victorian cities in England).

The presence of Harappan toilets connected to sewerage may be related to
some sort of awareness (whether metaphysical or empirical we do not know)
of the deadly danger posed by fecal-infected water supplies as causal agent of
diarrheal diseases. If cholera were already in existence (its history has yet to
be unravelled), fecal-infected water supplies would also transmit this disease.
The evolution in the last 40 years of two new cholera types (each more
deadly than the last) demonstrates the powerful Darwinian capabilities of
this disease.

In the Harappan empire (where cholera may or may not have been more
or less permanently present in the salty waters of the Arabian Gulf into
which the river Indus emptied – as it is today in the gulf into which the
Ganges empties), human behavior patterns may have encouraged the flourishing of another killing disease: bubonic plague. This may have merged
into pneumonic plague (with its 99 percent case mortality rate). Let us
explore these possibilities further.

Near Harappan city centers, wheaten-grain in large quantities was stored
in purpose-built structures. This practice might have assisted in the breeding
and maintenance of hordes of rats. Though rats with their fleas (if they
happen to be a susceptible form of flea) form only a part of the causal chain
of bubonic and pneumonic plague running from the bacillus *Yersinia pestis*
to humankind, the presence of these large urban grain storage bins, taken
in conjunction with the complete disappearance of the Harappan culture-
bearing elite around 1700 BCE, is "interesting."

From these and similar bits of evidence it can be suggested that the Indus
valley during the Harappan era *may* have been one of the places on planet
Earth where some of the major killing infectious diseases ("crowd diseases")

first jumped species (moving for instance from cows and chickens to humans) and then evolved through natural selection into human killers. Some of these diseases might have been maintained even after elite urban culture collapsed. This would have happened if several thousand ordinary people continued to live in market towns and farms not far from the old urban sites, thus ensuring that the Indus valley (as disease zone) was never entirely devoid of the human hosts of these infectious diseases.

As it happens, the Indus Valley was contiguous to the usual points of entry into the Indian subcontinent from ancient Persia and ancient Greece. Through piecing together bits of information, paleontologists and medical historians have begun to sort out when disease "x" and disease "y" were first reported in the Middle East or in southeastern Europe. Though the history of disease evolution is still very much in its infancy, preliminary conclusions tend to indicate a correlation between known inter-regional movements and the spread into Europe of new infectious killer diseases from India.

We know, for example, that troops recruited in the Indus Valley fought under the command of the Persians at Thermopylae in 480 BCE: along with the swords and shields they used against Athenians, they would have taken with them their contagious diseases. We also know that heretofore malaria-free Greek lands came to be regularly infected with that killing disease soon after Alexander the Great and his mutinous Greek soldiers passed through malarial regions on the way back west from northern India in 326 BCE. We also know that leprosy was unknown in Egypt before it was brought in by the Greeks from further east. Also unknown in Egypt, until brought in from India during the time of the Greeks, were chickens and their associated diseases.

Antecedents of Ayurvédic medicine

The Indian elite wisdom that had come into being by the beginning of our current era to form one of the Great Traditions in world medicine, Ayurvédic medicine, has a rather mixed ancestry. Some of the *written* (as opposed to orally transmitted) textual materials on which Ayurvédic medicine is based originally dated back to the first century CE. However, the first *extant* written sources – written on palm leaves – date only from the eighth century CE. These late surviving texts are heavily edited and contain a great deal of material which was added well after the first century CE. These additions were doubtless made in order to give the genuine (early CE) materials greater authority by providing them with roots that went back to the gods who were revered by the "respectable people" around 1600 BCE (see below). In its most developed forms, Ayurvédic medicine claims to be revealed truth brought from the land of the immortals.

Questionable though they are, claims that the beginnings of the Ayurvédic medical tradition date back some 3,500 years are of some interest. Many of them hinge on the posited existence of a powerful people who quite suddenly erupted into Indian history one, two, or three hundred years after the disappearance of the Harappan civilized elite. These people – of uncertain origin, but perhaps from central Asia – had a language they used for ritual purposes, called Sanskrit.

By about 1200 BCE the core myths of these Sanskrit-using peoples (who called themselves the "moral ones" or the "respectable people") had been put together in final form and were known as "the knowledge," the *veda*. In the course of the next 800 years, the "respectable people" (who quoted great chunks of the *veda* on ceremonial occasions) came to rule a hodge-podge of kingdoms and principalities that stretched across northern India and parts of today's Pakistan. Their largest concentration of settlement lay on the rich plains in the east, in Bengal, centered on the Ganges river system.

Important for understanding the conceptual bases which, much, much later, would underlie Ayurvédic medicine, were what the "respectable people," the "moral ones," regarded as the three pillars of their society. One pillar was the primacy given the knowledge orally transmitted over the generations in Sanskrit. The second was full acceptance of an authoritative priesthood (the Brahmins). The third pillar was acceptance of a hierarchical ordering of society, in nascent form, the Indian caste system with its several hundred variously defined gradations.

As will become apparent when we look at fully-fledged Ayurvédic medicine in more detail, until very late (after the third century CE) the Brahmins – the authoritative priesthood – regarded proto-medical doctors as lesser beings. Like the middle strata generally (merchants, traders and such like), proto-medical doctors regarded the making of a personal fortune as a legitimate life-time goal. It was not so regarded by the Brahmins.

Scholars who have studied the antecedents of Ayurvédic medicine tell us that among the "respectable people" in the period 800 to 600 BCE, two books of knowledge (*veda*) were called into being. Both dealt in one way or another with the causes of disease and possible cures. These were the *Rgveda c.* 800 BCE and the *Atharvaveda c.* 600 BCE.

In them, diseases that affected a person's inner workings were generally seen as being caused by one or another category of demons. In those cases, proto-medical professionals attempted to effect cures by ritually casting out the demons, not en masse, but one at a time, each demon being held responsible for each particular symptom.

Yet, during those same centuries (800–600 BCE), in attempting to deal with injuries to the exterior of the body which might be seen as being caused by natural forces, proto-professionals (especially in the *Atharvaveda* tradition) might use one or other medical plants or use an animal extract, for example, cow's urine. In the course of his activities, a proto-professional might also come into direct contact with the blood, fecal matter or urine of his patient: indeed it was standard diagnostic procedure to taste a bit of a patient's urine or fecal matter. This, medically-approved patient–healer exchange would have a long-term social impact.

Unmediated by other influences, as long as the *Rgveda* and the *Atharvaveda* alone set the tone, the Brahmin priestly caste regarded proto-professional medical men as ritually impure. It would be impossible for a Brahmin to sit down at the same table to share a meal with a person of this sort. Given this prejudice, it is not surprising that the books of knowledge that Brahmins generated in the next period, the so-called late Vedic period (after 600 BCE), had very little to say about disease or how to seek for cures: these were banned subjects.

The half-millennium after 600 BCE seems to have been one of great confusion. It appears that the Brahmins, with their near monopoly of "wisdom," were having difficulty in maintaining their grip over settled society. It seems, too, that all sorts of holy men and ascetics (some clothed, some naked) were roving about the countryside preaching messages about metaphysical and spiritual renewal: other ascetics preached the need to renounce all earthly pleasures.

At some point in the decades before Alexander the Great burst onto the scene, the son of a local ruler in the East, one Siddhartha Gautama (the Buddha), also began to wander around the countryside, preaching. In time, the Buddha's ascetic message attracted many followers. Though not in India itself (because of the effectiveness of Brahmin persecution), Buddhism became one of the major world religions.

The Buddha's teachings are generally agreed to have had a major impact on the making of Ayurvédic medicine. This, it can be argued, is *not* because these teachings were empirico-rational, but rather because they included all three sides of the triangle of healing. This, it will be remembered, consisted of the holy curer (the saint, or ascetic who was in touch with forces not entirely of this world), the sick one (the patient), and the disease itself.

According to the Buddha (looking at the first side of the triangle of healing), those of his followers who had the ability to alleviate or to cure diseases should accept no payment or reward for their services. Theirs was an act of charity which in itself confirmed the saintly character of the healer. Turning to the second and third sides of the triangle, the Buddha had interesting things to say about disease causation and the mind-sets of people who were sick. He held that inner causes of disease might involve an imbalance between the three bodily forces (*dosas*): "bile," "phlegm" and "wind," or their various combinations (I will say more about these un-Greek *dosas* in a moment).

Going on from there the Buddha also pointed out that perceptions of being sick might be caused by unpleasant experiences. Someone might come to feel sick if he had just been wrongly arrested for adultery, or if he had been roughed up and robbed by a thief, or if he had just escaped being bitten by a snake. Speaking in more general terms, the Buddha reminded people that they might also feel sick if they had just experienced a sudden change of seasons. On the other hand, they might feel sick if they had been sitting too long in one position, or standing too long. Moving then to the overtly metaphysical (and the concept of reincarnation), the Buddha said that sickness might come to a person because of the evil things he or she had done in a previous life.

The processes through which the Buddha's teachings on sickness, health and medicine were mediated through existing Hindu thought to become part of what, by early centuries of the current era, had become Ayurvédic medicine (India's medical mainstream), has not yet been clearly sorted out. However, one of the preconditions making possible the *full* integration of sometimes contradictory ideas into a coherent whole was the settling down of Indian society under the Gupta dynasty, beginning around 320 CE.

Based originally along the Ganges river system in central Bengal, in the course of the next few generations Gupta hegemony extended southward to the Coromandel coast and westward to the valley of the Indus (with its long-forgotten Harappan cities). Under this dynasty, India enjoyed social peace for nearly 200 years.

It would seem that it was during this long era of harmony that the Brahmins (the largely hereditary caste who preserved the authoritative wisdom from the past) agreed to compromise with members of the proto-medical profession. Each group, Brahmins and medics, agreed to live and let live, and to accept the permanence of the other.

As part of this compromise, Brahmins agreed that proto-physicians would be accepted as one of the categories of men of learning. They remained, of course, of a somewhat lower quality than the Brahmins themselves, but they had crossed the line and had almost made the grade into "respectability." In short, they were philosophers. This meant that it was accepted that their skills in curing were dependent on their deeper knowledge of the world of humankind and of the gods and of the inter-relationship between them. These intellectual achievements set medical practitioners firmly apart from quacks, charlatans, empirics and others who went around the countryside offering to cure people (for money) but who had no knowledge of the cosmos and how it related to humankind.

Marking the full acceptance of this compromise during the era of social harmony under the Gupta after 300 CE, the Brahmins finally accepted the *Rgveda* and the *Atharvaveda* (the magical, quasi-medical texts dating from the period 800–600 BCE) as part of the authentic corpus of sacred Hindu writings. With this, Ayurvédic medicine achieved full recognition among the authoritative priesthood. It was now part of a Great Tradition.

Ayurvédic medicine

Central to the maintenance of the Ayurvédic medical tradition was the existence of a well-defined cadre of medical professionals. And to sustain itself
intellectually, the profession also needed its own special books. Several of
the requisite compositions have survived. The oldest, dating from the early
centuries CE, is the *Caraka Samhita* (Caraka's *Compendium*) which seems to
have been written in northwestern India. The second, and slightly later
compendium, was by "Susruta" of Benares, (otherwise known as the *Susruta
Samhita*). The contrast between the precision of the dates I was able to
provide for medical manuals written in the Middle East (in Chapter 4) and
the vague guesstimates I give for Indian source compendia (based on the
best recent authorities) will be noted.

Much information about the training of medical professionals in the early
days is found in Caraka's *Compendium*. From this we learn that although
Brahmins had (by say 350 CE) come to accept medical doctors as worthy
beings, and sometimes permitted their own sons to join that profession,
they nevertheless didn't allow medical men to study the full range of *veda*
(the ancient wisdom). By restricting their training in this way, Brahmins
could safely continue to regard medical men as mere specialists, rather than
as fully fledged bearers of wisdom like themselves.

Other aspects of medical training also reflected priestly bias. Most apprentice medics studied under a senior family member who was already an
accredited doctor (among Brahmins, caste status was of course passed on
from father to son). And somewhat like that undertaken by apprentice
priests, medical apprenticeship began with an initiation ceremony in which
the apprentice swore that he would be fully obedient to his master and
that while living in his house he would cause no harm to any member of
the family. He also swore to remain chaste sexually and to eat no meat.
The apprentice was to dress modestly and be scrupulously honest.

Having learned to adopt the demeanor of a saintly healer, the apprentice
medico then set to the task of memorizing long passages of Caraka's
Compendium, Susruta's *Compendium* and other relevant works. This might
take several years. Then with this great corpus of memorized wisdom in
mind, the apprentice, who had at last become a fully fledged doctor, would
be in a position to address the problems of individual patients.

According to the accepted formula, consultation would begin with the
doctor asking the patient to describe his symptoms and why he felt sick.
Elements in the patient's narrative would remind the doctor of analogous
situations he had memorized from one of the great medical compendiums.
Putting the two parts of the dialogue together (the present and the past),
he would prescribe an appropriate treatment or therapeutic drug (more on
this below).

Lying at the heart of the mental world of Hindu medicine was the philosophical conviction that there was a fundamental division between those

things that were permanent, fixed and unchanging, and those things that were subject to change. Among humankind (the subject matter of medicine), the element that was immutable was the "soul": it of course was male. Constituting the other half of the discourse, the element that was in a state of constant flux during the life-cycle events of birth, babyhood, youth, adulthood and old age was the "body": it represented the feminine principle.

In order to more fully understand why Ayurvédic medicine had no interest in conducting empirical study of the human anatomy by hacking up semi-dead convicts as Herophilus of Alexandria had done around 270–260 BCE, let us explore the Hindu mental world further.

According to Caraka's and Susruta's medical compendiums (written three or four hundred years after Herophilus's time) the "body" contained three forces or *dosas* (which it is quite wrong to translate as Greek-style "humors" following the Hippocratic Corpus). These *dosas* consisted of "wind," "bile" and "phlegm": each of these terms contained within itself a multitude of meanings.

Basically, "wind" was the life force which caused movement within the human body, male or female. Working from its headquarters in the heart (the central organ of the body), "wind" pushed the sustenance (food) that had gone into the stomach through its various stages, forming itself into fat and muscle, and as blood and bone: (these are four of the seven vital tissues of which the body consisted). At each stage in the purification process of creating vital tissue, waste products were secreted or eliminated. Coming at the end of the long process, and affecting only a small residue, was the marrow of the bone (the sixth vital tissue) which was further purified to form the highest and purest substance, semen, the seventh vital tissue. Surplus semen was stored in a man's heart, and among its other attributes it represented "light." In a virginal young woman, "light" (metaphysically injected into her fabric) was what gave brightness to her face and eyes, and bounce to her body.

"Wind," "bile" and "phlegm" (each with their own special functions) worked their way through the human "body" by way of a complex system of channels: each pore on the skin represented the terminal point of one of these channels. Disease was caused when one or other of the three *dosas* overflowed its own channel, or became blocked in its channel. Reflecting this dualism, one of the basic definitions of *dosa* was "vice" or "defect." The role of the physician was, of course, to determine which of the *dosas* ("wind," "bile," "phlegm") was not performing its allotted tasks, and to sort out how to restore an orderly flow.

I have already said something about the importance of the "heart" (*mahat*). Within this schema, *mahat* was analogous to the king's palace. In addition to being the seat of the human soul (the immutable, male force), *mahat* also contained the mind (and source of human consciousness) which sent out directions to all other elements in the body. It (rather than the human brain as understood by modern science) was the command center of the system.

Very much like the ancient Egyptians (with whom they may never have had direct contact, despite the presence of Middle Kingdom trade goods in India), practitioners of Ayurvédic medicine before and after 300 CE did not regard the human brain as having any particular physiological or medically interesting function. Neither were they interested in the nerves connecting the spinal column to the brain. Yet, despite the absence in their world view of brains and of central nervous systems, Ayurvéda practitioners possessed what was for them (thanks to their metaphysical schema) a complete and satisfying explanation of the workings of the cycle of human existence.

In this, their ideas about the processes of human reproduction are of some interest. In Ayurvédic medical thinking (set forth in Caraka's *Compendium*), a male deposited his semen in the body of a woman. This semen was, at one and the same time, an element of his own "soul," and the "soul" of the yet to be born who would be nourished in the womb of the mother. Both "souls" were part of the unchanging, infinite permanence. Both souls were, of course, male; human women only existed in order to assist in the creation of male children. Once equipped with "soul" by its father, the child in the womb derived its "body" from its mother; she gave it an essence of her own heart. During this period of exchange, the pregnant woman's health and life-chances were precarious; this was seen as the natural order of things.

The professional grouping that specialized in knowing what the natural order was, in as much as it affected human beings, consisted of the Ayurvédic practitioners. As the ones who knew what "the rules" were, they were scrupulously careful to keep their distance from quacks, charlatans and the like who had no specialized professional training in the metaphysics of medicine.

In their consultations with clients, Ayurvédic practitioners called to mind the "rules" that by analogy might apply to the medical and psychic problems from which their clients suffered. From a purely medical view they realized (and helped the client to understand) that change and decay was part of the normal human cycle. Men and women who were past, say, the age of 30, could not expect their *dosas* to flow as regularly and as smoothly as those found in a younger person. Yet, in as much as the self-professed purpose of Ayurvédic medicine was to enable people to live to a healthy old age (variously defined, perhaps 80 or 120 years) a practitioner's duty was to assist their clients to restore the good ordering of their *dosa* appropriate to their age, lifestyle, and status. Practitioners insisted that, contrary to the claims of patent medicine dealers, there *was* no one standard remedy that could be applied to everyone in all circumstances.

In the nature of things, Ayurvédic practitioners (as highly educated men, some closely related by blood to Brahmins) were in great demand among royal personages in Indian courtly palaces. They were also in great demand among the merchant princes in Gujarat who, by the fourteenth century, were laying down the regional foundations of sophisticated Indian capitalism, with ties to Cairo and to China. Yet, in their professional capacities, practitioners remained somewhat ambivalent about the sort of life-style that was most conducive to a healthy life and old age. They were not convinced that the highly formalized behavioral patterns and rich food found in a royal court were healthy. Indeed, they had good reason to admire the (idealized) mind-set of simple peasant cultivators.

Following ancient teachings (not least those of the Buddha, though they would not admit to this), Ayurvédic practitioners believed that many diseases (in effect, the dysfunctioning of the *dosa*) were caused by a person's perception that he/she was being unnaturally constrained and repressed. This feeling was most commonly felt by urban sophisticates whose life-style was contrary to "nature." In a proper, ordered existence, as found among peasant cultivators, men, women and children literally followed the prompting of nature. If they needed to defecate, they did so; to urinate, they did so; to release gas by farting or belching, they did so. Among the peasantry, performance of these natural functions in full public view was not a cause of shame. As practitioners knew, to feel shame, or embarrassment (as urban sophisticates did), would lead to pent up feelings and to disorder among the *dosa*.

In order to restore the proper functioning of a person's *dosa* an Ayurvédic practitioner first perhaps resorted to psychological counseling, following the many injunctions found in the Sanskrit medical compendium by Caraka (of northwestern India) and Susruta (of the holy city of Benares). Then, if it were necessary to go beyond this, the practitioner would prescribe one or other type of physical treatments.

Interestingly enough, although there is a lengthy chapter about the role of surgery in the early CE *Compendium* by Susruta (telling a practitioner how to remove gall stones, cataracts, suturing wounds together and the like), all later Ayurvédic practitioners seem to have stayed clear of performing surgical operations. Modern logic suggests that most people who, in the early centuries, had come under a surgeon's knife died in the process. Thus, to do surgery, under the guise of Ayurvédic medicine, threatened the survival of the profession as a whole. Fortunately there were other alternatives at hand.

Ayurvédic medicine was known for the great emphasis it placed on proper diet; one that was appropriate to the circumstances, life-style and age of a patient. Among the dietary prescriptions it frequently recommended were broths. These would consist of a meat stock which had been boiled down, concentrating its vital essences. In some cases, another meat would then be added to this concentrate and the whole boiled down again; this process might be repeated several times. In the case of a prince, with a large hunting preserve at his disposal, the first meat might have been that of an ox, and the second (added in the second cooking) that of the heart of a lion or tiger. But, given that cows were sacred to Hindus and that lion meat was not considered fit for human consumption, the patient would be told that he was eating a broth made from goat or some other socially acceptable beast.

Emerging from this example are three important points. First, since an Ayurvédic practitioner knew what "the rules" were, he was at liberty to break them if circumstances required. One constraint he had overridden in the cited example was his student oath never to tell a lie (he had in fact lied to the patient about the contents of the broth). The second rule he had overridden was to prescribe cow meat (sacred and forbidden to Hindus) but only in normal circumstances; here "normal" was defined by the practitioner. The third point I want to draw is the very obvious analogy between the boiling down processes, leading to refined essences, and the work done in the human body by "wind" as it drove raw foods in the stomach through the various stages of purification (and waste extraction) to become one of the seven vital tissues.

Another important point about Ayurvédic dietary prescriptions should be mentioned. As found in the compendiums by Caraka and Susruta, the prescription is very often *not* inserted by mouth, orally. Instead, in more than 100 examples, it was inserted through the media of an enema, through the anus. As we saw, in ancient Egypt, one of the principal physicians at a pharaoh's court was the guardian of the king's anus. Whether or not there was any connection between these two phenomena, so different in time and space, it is impossible to say.

Unani Tibb: Hellenistic medicine

Ayurvédic medicine survived the coming of Mughal rule in the early sixteenth century. Initially conquered in and after 1505 by Babur, the Muslim ruler of Afghanistan and the Punjab, by mid-century the Indian subcontinent was unified under the benign rule of Babur's descendant, Akbar (1556–1605). Among the pillars sustaining Akbar's long rule was toleration for all religious groupings within his empire. Though not strictly speaking "people of the book" of the sort the Prophet Muhammad (in the Qur'an) had enjoined his followers to respect, Akbar nevertheless regarded Hindus as bearers of a worthy civilization.

With the coming of Mughal rule, sizeable numbers of Unani Tibb practitioners (called *hakims*) moved southward from Afghanistan and eastward from the Punjab to settle down in India. As we saw in Chapter 4, *hakims* were Muslims who followed the medical tradition created in the Islamic world by Ibn Sina through his *Canon*. Working within the perimeters of that great tradition, they understood full well that the practitioners of Ayurvédic medicine (called *vaids*) lived in a mental world different from their own. Nevertheless, at a time when diseases were generally only overcome by nature's own healing processes (encouraged perhaps by good counseling), *hakims* recognized that *vaids* were as competent as they were themselves.

Folk medicine

In 1700, when the population of the Indian subcontinent hovered around 180 million, it is likely that 95 percent of its people lived in scattered clusters of villages, rather than in large urban centers or in princely compounds. It seems likely too that relatively few of these rural people had much contact with urban-based practitioners of Ayurvéda or of Unani Tibb medicine. Instead, in time of personal sickness, or when their village was threatened by an epidemic, they had recourse to a carefully thought-out schedule of actions appropriate to the occasion.

Some of the concepts incorporated into village medicine – for example, the great symbolic importance given to semen and the role of dietary restrictions – had close parallels in Ayurvédic medicine. Others, however, were far removed from the intellectualized metaphysics that underlay that great tradition or the rationalism that underlay Unani Tibb medicine.

Within a village's medical schema (each slightly different from that of neighboring villages) there was a graded hierarchy of sickness causal agents. "Accidental" conditions were seen as being brought on by carelessly performed everyday activities or perhaps by a dietary mistake. Too many "cold" foods (green vegetables, milk) could lead to a flu-like condition; too many "hot" foods (meat, spicy foods) could lead to a feverish condition. From this it followed that a fever was best confronted by withholding food until it subsided.

Within the perceptual world of the village, another cause of personal sickness was "pollution." A male might be "polluted" if he saw a woman's menstrual blood. Or he might be "polluted" if he saw a newborn infant's severed umbilical cord, or the caul which had surrounded the infant in its mother's womb. A person might also be "polluted" by coming into contact with a human corpse. Removing the mess which had brought on the "pollution" was done by a member of the "untouchable" caste who, by definition, was immune to its effects. Among people of higher status "pollution" could be countered by ceremonial bathing.

Moving up the causal scale, but still dealing with sickness among individuals, village medicine held that serious complaints were caused by behavioral transgressions, either in this life, or in a previous existence. Hacking coughs and spitting up blood for instance might be caused by one or another form of sexual misconduct. Similarly, splitting headaches might be caused by anti-social behavior. The local healer, who was called in to deal with a case (a sick young woman for example), generally worked in tandem with village elders. This meant that the healer already knew what the cause of the complaint was without being told by the sufferer. Thus, the coming of "disease" acted as a tool for social control by elders upon the young, and by senior men upon women.

More dramatic was the response thought appropriate to the coming of major epidemic diseases, such as smallpox. In such circumstances, the village recognized that the disease disaster (either present or imminent) was being sent against them by an irate goddess – Sitala, or Miriamma – whom they had failed to propitiate by regular corporate worship. Recognizing that the goddess was both the "cause" of the disaster, as well as the media through which they needed to work to clear it away, they organized elaborate corporate rituals.

Very often, at the center of this ritual was a procession of the entire community, marching behind a mock-up statue of the goddess. After touring all the quarters of the village to gather up her essences there, they marched out of the built-up area, hoping that they had persuaded her to leave them in peace and to move on to the next village. Alternatively, the village would attempt to appease Sitala by welcoming her into their midst. When a child or adult fell sick with smallpox, they would crowd into the sickroom and congratulate each other for the fact that their obscure village had been honored by the presence of the goddess.

Yet, emerging from the village world in which such things happened was an empirically based procedure which was used to prevent outbreaks of smallpox. Perhaps even before the seventeenth century, barbers and other non-standard health workers went around the villages inducing mild cases of smallpox among children. Through the processes of variolation or *inoculation* (scratching a bit of attenuated smallpox matter into the skin or putting it up the nose), their intention was to provide the children with life-long immunity against the disease.

In the nature of things in pre-British times, no statistical data was generated to testify to the success of their efforts. Then, in the 1860s and early 1870s statistics began to be kept by medical doctors brought in by the British rulers of the land. Finding that there was much less smallpox among adults in Bengal than in other parts of India, they occasionally admitted that this was perhaps because these adults had been inoculated as children. However, as part of their new-found conviction that real knowledge in any field was a monopoly of the West (an attitude much strengthened by events in the late 1850s – the Great Rebellion), the British outlawed inoculation and insisted that Indian children should be vaccinated in the way that British children were, following the teachings of Edward Jenner (d. 1823).

Much to their annoyance however, British medical authority found that Hindu parents often refused to have their children *vaccinated* with serum derived from cows, forgetting that for Hindus cows were a sacred animal that should not be harmed. British authority was also annoyed to find that many Indians realized that vaccination (à la Jenner) did *not* provide lifetime immunity in the way that inoculation did. Yet the British insisted, that because they were British, they knew best.

Conclusion

The subcontinent of India was certainly not a disease-free paradise in the early eighteenth century on the eve of the weakening of the Mughal Empire through the actions of regional Hindu and Muslim princelings, followed later in the century by conquest by the armies of the British East India Company. Yet, because the physical environment occupied by 95 percent of the population was rural and because village groupings were able to move away from any place which they perceived was infected by lethal disease agents, it seems likely that whole regions were seldom devastated by mass killing epidemics.

This situation changed for the worse after 1757 with the establishment of British Company rule, first in Bengal, then, through diplomacy and military conquests, over the subcontinent as a whole. As part of their *Pax Britannia* and what they regarded as a necessary part of the process of modernization (making Indians into obedient tax-paying servants of Empire), the new rulers of the land forcibly stabilized and settled whole populations. They also deliberately undermined the fabric of every village society and destroyed the moral core of the old property-holding classes. After the opening of the Suez Canal in 1869 massively increased the scale of Indian investment returns coming into the hands of Britain's financial elite, continuing disruptive ecological and psychological interventions in India were followed by increasingly destructive waves of epidemic disease (see Chapter 9).

Further reading

Most English-language writings on the history of Ayurvédic medicine have been heavily tainted by Orientalism (Indians as "Other"). Invented, much twisted history of Ayurvédic medicine before 1757 was also created by successive generations of Indian nationalists who felt compelled to prove that Indians had long since invented the Germ Theory and similar modern concepts. Bearing these caveats in mind, some useful insights can be found in Kenneth Zysk, *Asceticism and Healing in Ancient India* (New York: Oxford University Press, 1991) and Dominik Wujastyk, "Indian Medicine" in William Bynum and Roy Porter (eds) *Companion Encyclopedia of the History of Medicine* (London: Routledge, 1993). A preliminary report on ongoing research at the India Office (London) on the collapse of disease control measures in India following the opening of the Suez Canal is at the Cambridge University history website: www.historyandpolicy.org/.

Chapter 6

Medicine and disease in China

Concepts and practices from
c. 1900 BCE to 1840 CE

Introduction

Learned medicine has existed in China for several thousand years. In this chapter our concern is with its history from earliest times until the Chinese Imperial regime faltered in the face of British invaders in and after 1840. Just here however it is useful first to remind ourselves of the pivotal nature of the events of the 1840s and 1850s and of the massive impact they have had on the writing of medical history.

In the course of the Opium Wars of 1839–42 and 1858–60, British and Sepoy troops from India forced the fiercely reluctant Chinese government to agree to import huge quantities of opium, the hallucinatory drug grown in India, and to pay for it with silver. In this triangular round-about way, Great Britain's huge negative trade imbalance with India (which wanted nothing England produced) came to be off-set by Chinese silver. This use of armed force upon a Non-western land to ensure England's own economic stability and growth was a policy cut out from the same cloth as was England's seventeenth- and eighteenth-century policy of promoting the trade in Black African slaves to the New World.

In both cases, what is particularly important from our point of view is that the triumph of Western armaments over less aggressive Non-western peoples meant that Western agents thereafter would scornfully depreciate the medical practices of the victim societies, claiming that they were based on raw superstition. In the case of a China which came to be haunted by medical missionaries of the evangelical bent of mind, this Western prejudice became all-pervasive. Its long-term presence is one of the major reasons why currently, for the period before 1840, the literature available to Western historians of medicine who do not read Chinese is dominated by discussions of highly intellectualized *theory*, far removed from anything that could be construed to be "superstition": very little is said about actual practice.

However, by approaching the question of "practice" from another direction – using the findings of historic demographers – we arrive at interesting conclusions. We discover that as of 1700–50 CE, the health status of the 30 to

40 million people living in the principal cities in the Yangzi Delta (Shanghai, Suzhou, Hangzhou) and in rural areas around about, was rather *better* than it was at the time among the same-sized population of France. Statistics show that Chinese people lived longer, despite the fact that most of the debilitating and infectious diseases (including venereal syphilis) found in the hexagon of France around 1750 were also found in the Yangzi Delta region. We of course do not know whether longevity depended on the presence of medical doctors and other practitioners, or whether it depended on a standard of living which was generally higher in the Yangzi Delta than it was in any of the cultural heartlands of Europe during its age of Enlightenment.

In writing the history of Chinese medicine, one of the greatest barriers is the difficulty of the Chinese language itself. Like Chinese civilization, it has been in continuous existence for 3,500 years. However, many of its several thousand written symbols have variant, sometimes contradictory, meanings: some meanings have drifted over time. Thus, even for native-born Chinese historians, the task of learning the written language is formidable. Among Westerners, long-years of instruction have only rarely led to complete command even of existing Chinese scholarship, to say nothing of the ability to read ancient texts.

As a result, most of what native-born Chinese medical historians have written – using the scholarly minimum of 8,000 characters – has yet to be translated into a European language. Looking in the other direction, and taking into account normal inter-cultural and inter-disciplinary time-lags, it also means that recent trends in Euro-American medico-cultural history have yet to have much impact on writings in the field in China.

Five initial keys to understanding

Key 1

The easiest way for Western students of history to tackle Chinese medical ideas and practices as they evolved between *c.* 1900 BCE and 1840 CE (a period of 3,740 years) is to accept that Chinese thought patterns were entirely different than those found in dominant medical circles in the West – especially after the work of Koch in the 1880s (see Chapter 9).

Key 2

In pre-modern China, just as in pre-modern India, the task of establishing standard medical-related interpretations and texts was undertaken largely by philosophers and other scholars intent on building up grand systems which explained everything in the universe. Given that purpose, they did not attempt to build systems based on knowledge of the organs in an actual human body. Instead, using the insights of speculative philosophy, they assigned essentially mythic functions to concepts for which they used the names "heart," "liver," "spleen," "lungs" and "kidneys." Though there were a few exceptions over the three millennia, most speculative Chinese medical systems omitted to mention the human brain, as concept. It was perhaps mere coincidence that they shared this trait with ancient Egyptian medicine and with Ayurvédic medicine in India.

Key 3

This takes us again to the discipline of philosophy and its sub-discipline, logic. Using insights from these fields, it is clear that there was a major difference in the standard conceptual patterning found among Chinese literate elites from that civilization's beginnings until almost the present, compared to the standard conceptual patterning found in the West from the nineteenth century CE onwards. Let me explain.

In the West, educated people often think in terms of a system of logic formalized by the German philosopher G. W. F. Hegel (1770–1831). Hegelian logic holds that each idea or situation (the *thesis*) generates its opposite (*antithesis*) and that the two come together to form a *synthesis*, which in turn becomes the new *thesis* which generates its antithesis and so on. This movement of ideas (or situations) through time ("the march of history" or "the march of God in history"), constitutes progress in the nineteenth-century sense of the word.

But in "traditional" Chinese medical thought, nothing like that existed. Instead, any of the leading medical or medical-related ideas that could be taken to constitute a *thesis* dating from the formative period of Chinese medicine, 260 BCE to 220 CE, was commented upon, and perhaps manipulated in the course of the next 2,000 years, but (and this is the really important point) it was never entirely rejected. Thus, though some frail attempts at synthesis and weeding out were made during the high-tide of intellectual activity that occurred around 1650–1750 CE in the Lower Yangzi region, these attempts came to nothing. Years later, the original ancient conceptual core (*thesis*) from 260 BCE to 220 CE was still being trotted out in the expectation that it would be regarded as insightful and useful.

This was obviously quite different from the situation in the Middle East where, in the early eleventh century CE, all existing medical ideas were synthesized into a single corpus by Ibn Sina. For several centuries, it was also entirely different from the situation in western Europe where in and after the late eleventh century, Ibn Sina's *Canon* was taken to represent all the best of the medical knowledge of the past.

However in the mid-eighteenth century, in Edinburgh (then a key center of the Enlightenment) there was a revival of interest in the fifth- to fourth-century BCE Hippocratic notion that diseases were caused by a miasma, an agency coming in from the outside. Ironically, this process of reviving an ancient idea (which among some eighteenth- and early nineteenth-century medical thinkers replaced Romano-Greek Galenic *humoral* ideas) was not dissimilar to the Chinese medical intellectual practice of keeping a range of disparate ideas from all periods in active circulation.

Key 4

During the last 2,500 years (since the time of the Han dynasty, 206 BCE–220 CE), those involved in Chinese medicine, as health care providers or as theorizers, have been intensely *individualistic*. This has had a very considerable impact on the development of the medical field. Let us first turn to the itinerants and their apprentices who (along with local curers of both sexes) served the health care needs of the peasant population out in the countryside.

Here, there seems to be no question but that each itinerant curer competed openly with all others for the custom of would-be patients. Each claimed to have some unique insight, or some uniquely efficient all-purpose way to exorcize demons, or a curative combination of drugs that could cure all illnesses, which was available, for a price. This situation was not perhaps unexpected.

However, of greater consequence for future developments, a somewhat similar situation prevailed among the *literate* medical elite. Here, each individual writer was intent on making his (gender intended) mark on the world by coming up with a slightly different interpretation of existing medical-related knowledge. In consequence, several more or less persuasive interpretations co-existed at the same time, none of which was able permanently to supercede the rest. Really innovative work was not encouraged. As a result, within Chinese intellectual circles, nothing like say the Germ Theory (of the 1860s onward, Robert Koch, Louis Pasteur) could win through to create what was in effect in the West, a new field of human endeavor, modern scientific medicine.

Key 5

In China, during the 3,740 year period (civilizational beginnings to 1840) revealed in surviving texts, there was often a fruitful bottom-up as well as a top-down exchange between itinerant health care providers and the philosopher-physicians who wrote learned treatises on medical-related issues.

A good example is the ancient conviction (in place by 1900 BCE) that disease was sent in by an *outside* force, a demon, and that it could be expelled by exorcism or other rituals. In popular medicine, this idea remained well entrenched until the twentieth century CE. The case was not much different within learned medicine. At least until the mid-eighteenth century CE, well-known medico-philosophers wove the concept of "demon" as disease-cause-to-be-cleansed-away-by-exorcism into textual interpretations of what actually caused disease and what should be done about it.

By way of contrast, in the medieval and early modern West no respectable physician would ever admit that he had anything to learn from itinerant practitioners, all of whom he regarded as fakes and charlatans. Similarly, from the late fourteenth century onwards it is unlikely that many doctors with university degrees thought in terms of demons as disease causal agents, except perhaps in the case of madness.

General considerations in Chinese medical history

A question of central concern to any historian of medicine is to ask what impact a given system of medicine had upon the recipient population. But in dealing with China we have to rephrase the question to read "systems" of medicine, since no one system ever prevailed.

One general consideration in writing the history of Chinese medicine before 1840 is the need to understand that centuries-long periods of chaos were no less productive in the creation of new "medical" philosophical ideas, than were long periods of internal harmony and peace. Prime examples are the "Warring States Period" (403–221 BCE) and the chaotic late Song period which preceded the eventual re-unification of China under foreign Mongol rule (the dynasty in place between 1279–1368 CE).

This again contrasts with the situation in Europe. There, after the disintegration of the Roman Empire in the West in the late fourth and early fifth centuries, nothing resembling a medical profession (based on literacy and knowledge of the Galenic tradition) existed at all. Six hundred years later, in the late eleventh and early twelfth centuries, the foundation stones on which the European medical profession would eventually be built in the high middle ages had to be re-introduced anew from centers of Muslim learning. But in China, a learned medical profession has been in continuous existence from earliest times until the present.

The second general consideration in Chinese medical history is the need to place developments fully within their immediate temporal, social and intellectual contexts. Particularly in the formative centuries between 260 BCE to 220 CE, it was elements in this overall Chinese context (especially in the fields of metaphysics and philosophy) that provided the basis for the creation of the analogies and metaphors which in later periods would serve as guiding principles in Chinese medicine.

The formative period: core concepts

Coming out of the formative era of Chinese medical history which lasted until the end of the Han Dynasty (220 CE) were the several sets of concepts which from then onwards would be mixed and intermixed in a great variety of ways to form newer systems. At the risk of oversimplification, these conceptual sets can be divided into three general groups.

The first grouping was the most ancient, and was entirely magical. It held that disease was nearly always caused by an evil *outside* force, such as a hateful neighbor or an irate ancestor whose shrine had been neglected. In one way or another, this outside force or influence had to be driven out of the sick person's body. These magical ideas continued to be accepted by a great swath of the population well into the twentieth century.

The second grouping of conceptual sets might also be regarded as magical, though specialists would prefer to use the term "speculative philosophical." Extremely sophisticated, even in its most rudimentary form, this conceptual set was based on the mystic idea that there was a precise (if not always clearly intelligible) relationship, or correspondence, between the known universe at large (the macrocosm) and the sick individual (the microcosm).

As perfected during the Han period, systems of Systematic Correspondences maintained that "correct" behavior in all things would ensure good health. Ill-health was caused by overstepping the bounds of what was proper. It was the duty of the physician to sort out which "bounds" had been overstepped and to prescribe remedies that would restore the proper balance which would again lead to good health.

With their emphasis on correct behavior by the microcosm (the individual) so as not to run foul of the rules of the macrocosm, the universe, otherwise known as the "well-ordered Imperial regime," systems of Systematic Correspondences stressed political and ethical conformity. Their ideal human subject was a mandarin, a civil servant in the Imperial bureaucracy. Later, we will look at Systematic Correspondences' many links with the ethical system known as Confucianism.

The third grouping of conceptual sets (anciently established, but flexible over time) perversely *rejected* the idea that a balanced and cautious life-style would always insure good health. Instead it held that violent loutish people, crude, rugged individualists who took what they wanted from the sickly, stunted poor might enjoy the robust good health that moral people sought after.

This conceptual set had at least the potential of looking at disease as a morally-neutral entity that could affect anybody (whatever their moral condition) which could be countered by taking an appropriate drug and perhaps by undergoing a massage or acupuncture and moxibustion (defined below). Why this third conceptual set (with its perhaps all too obvious – hence misleading – parallels with modern Western biomedicine) failed to win its way through to supremacy over the other two remains one of the unsolved mysteries of Chinese medical history.

"Classical" Chinese medicine

The making of Chinese medicine was a dynamic, irregular process. Thus we find that the era of the Shang and the Zhou (a long period of steady accretion of magical thought about how to keep the spirits of the ancestors happy) was suddenly replaced by an era of startling innovation. This was the late Warring States and the Han periods (c. 260 BCE–220 CE) which saw the creation of what is now known as Classical Chinese medicine. As a pre-condition for this development, it is also the period which saw the end of localistic feudal chaos, and which, under the Han Dynasty, saw the first creation of a centralized, bureaucratic state staffed by civil servants, mandarins, who came into their positions not by inheritance, but through passing a rigorous set of examinations.

Historians, working with archaeologists and linguists, have been able to give relatively precise dates to the creation of the varied strands in core groupings of medical concepts (for instance, *yin-yang* and the Five Phases (*wuxing*) – defined below) that came fully into being during this formative period. In doing this they have been able to use several actual documents written more than 2,000 years ago. By way of contrast, as we saw in Chapter 5, in India historians only have access to ancient texts through the medium of edited copies made up after 800 CE, several centuries after the originals had been written.

In 1975, archaeologists discovered and opened three tombs that had been closed in 165 BCE. These long-sealed tombs contained medical manuscripts written 50 to 100 years earlier. Among them was one of the earliest known copies of the *Inner Classic of the Yellow Sovereign*. In modern times, ever since the eighteenth century CE, the *Inner Classic* has been considered one of the two core books in Classical Chinese medicine.

The *Inner Classic* is a collection of essays written at different times, by different authors, some of whom contradicted what older authors in the collection had said. The beauty of the 1975 *Inner Classic* tomb-find was that it hadn't been messed around with during the Song Dynasty period (960–1279 CE) when tidy-minded bureaucrats severely edited many *Inner Classic* collections earlier known to modern scholars.

Historians who were at ease with ancient Chinese script sorted through the 1975 tomb-find, and through critical reading were able to put the *Inner Classic* essays in roughly chronological order. They then decided that the prototype and nearly mature *yin-yang* and Five Phases material they had in hand could not have evolved from earlier Chinese medical thought. Instead it must either have been brought in from the outside (but from where? from which outside?) or been the work of a cadre of self-taught geniuses who had not been shaped intellectually by previous Chinese medical writing.

The revolutionary breakthrough first exemplified in the oldest essays in the *Inner Classic* is that the health or illness situation of individual men is not caused by malevolent demons or ancestors. Instead, it is caused by happenings in the natural world which can be studied and comprehended by mankind, using *human reason*.

Setting the tone for nearly everything that came later, this stage in the making of the medical revolution which put "human reason" at its center was clearly under the direction of intellectuals who were *not* "medical doctors" in any meaningful sense of the word. Though hard evidence for this from other sources has yet to emerge, it appears that during the late Warring States and Han period, medical practitioners who actually touched clients in the course of consultations (for example, while taking their pulse – *mai*) did not enjoy as high a status as did desk-bound scholarly theoreticians, philosophers, and metaphysicians. From this it becomes apparent that the revolution in medical theory that glorified "human reason" was produced by scholars of just this sort – speculative philosophers. If involved in its conceptualization at all, practicing medical men (who had first-hand knowledge of actual human bodies) were kept on only as subordinate consultants.

In its early days (hinted at in the oldest essays in the *Inner Classic*), the Medicine of Systematic Correspondences was relatively simple. Then, in characteristic Chinese fashion, over the generations as student-disciples succeeded their masters and improved upon, or altered what the old men had said, it became more and more complex. Indeed, one could almost speak of an interrelated network of *systems*, rather than of a single system. In the end (by around 215 BCE – the date of the most recent text in the *Inner Classic* tomb-find of 1975) the Medicine of Systematic Correspondences had already become a complex intellectual maze in which one could wander around for years without ever coming to a definite conclusion about cause and effect relationships that would hold good in all times and all places.

But one should bear in mind that this was perhaps precisely what practicing medical doctors at the time wanted. Hired by wealthy mandarins and gentry who were intensely individualistic and jealous of their colleagues, a practitioner's business was to diagnose his client's illnesses. Provided with a complex of sometimes mutually contradictory medical correspondences, he could pick and choose which of them was most appropriate to the case at hand. Except in time of an epidemic disease from which everyone suffered, no client wanted to be diagnosed as having exactly the same afflictions as did his friends and rivals. Given this societal context (in which individualism was prized), the complexity of the many *yin-yang* categories was an ideal diagnostic tool.

Now for some definitions. In the making of *yin-yang* categories, philosophers had noted that in the natural world there is generally a division into two: night and day, the shady side of a hill (*yin*) and the sunny side of the hill (*yang*). From this it followed that everything connected with the human body could also be divided into a *yin* and a *yang*.

In earlier treatises the two-fold division sufficed. However, in later writings (discovered in the 1975 tomb-finds), the *yin* and the *yang* had both been subdivided into three. All of what were taken to be the body's major organs were attached to one or other of these six divisions. Thus, the small intestine and urinary bladder were credited with the qualities of the Major *yang*; the large intestine and stomach with the qualities of *yang* Brilliance. The Major *yin* was associated with the lungs and spleen, the Minor *yin* with the heart and kidneys, the Ceasing *yin* with the "heart-enclosing network" and liver. For their part the gallbladder and so-called triple burner were associated with the qualities of the Minor *yang*: the "triple burner" corresponded to no human organ known to modern medicine.

Also differing from what modern medical men and scientists regard as parts of the actual Natural World are the so-called "Five Phases" (*wuxing*). In Chinese thought the term refers to five "materials" that are in the *process* of interaction with one of the other four. Historians who think of their discipline as the study of societies undergoing change (societies in process), and geologists who think of the earth (with its shifting tectonic plates) as "process" should have no difficulty in understanding the concept of "process" when applied in the Chinese medical fashion to the five "materials" – water, fire, metal, wood and earth. None of these names should be taken as applying to actual substances (or phenomena, in the case of "fire") as we now know them.

In Chinese medical logic, each of these five "materials" could either over-come one of the other materials, or (since process can be a two-way thing) bring into being (generate) one of the other materials. Thus, as examples of overcoming, it was metaphorically said that earth blocks the passage of water (as in a dam) and that water extinguishes fire. Working in the other direction, it was metaphorically said that water brought into being wood (plants and trees need water in order to grow) and that wood brings into being fire (wood is fuel for fire).

Integral to the Medicine of Systematic Correspondences, each of the Five Materials in Process (the Five Phases, *wuxing*) was held to be mystically connected with appropriate parts of the natural environment, the universe, which constituted the macrocosm. Moving from macrocosm to microcosm (individual persons), each of the Five Materials in Process was also identified with an appropriate part of the human body.

According to one ancient interpretation, the human "spleen" was identified with the qualities of "earth"; the "liver" with that of wood; and the "lungs" with that of "metal." Thus, for diagnostic purposes, a practitioner would consider that a "disease agent" that moved from the "liver" to the "lungs" was less dangerous ("wood" poses no threat to "metal") than was a "disease agent" that moved from "spleen" to "liver" (since earth's son, "metal," cuts wood). Indeed, according to this diagnostic system, any disease moving from spleen to liver was likely to prove fatal.

As they ripened to maturity in around 220 CE (end of Han) the closely interrelated, sometimes contradictory, networks of thought that constituted the Medicine of Systematic Correspondences contained other elements of interest. One held that the heart, the spleen and the other principal organs were all connected to other parts of the body (and especially to the skin, with its all-important 84,000 pores) either by one network, or by five separate networks of "conduits." Thus, any disease agent (i.e. "wind" *feng*) that came in through the ends of individual hairs on the scalp would go down to the "kidneys" and cause severe problems. "Kidneys" (the chief organ in a complex system) would also be adversely affected by rotting teeth. Though the literature sometimes expressed interest in "conduits," the visible veins and arteries (as we would call them) on the back of human hands and at the inside of the wrists, it was never clearly stated of what these "conduits" consisted.

Then, too, there was lack of agreement in sorting out the differing functions of the two liquid-like or mystic substances that were carried back and forth between the extremities (toes, fingers, ends of each hair on the head). One of these substances was blood; the other was *qi* (also known as *pneuma*).

Just as is the case with the Five Materials in Process, so too *qi* has *no* meaningful parallel in fifth- and fourth-century BCE Hippocratic Greek medical thought. According to Paul Unschuld, in literal translation *qi* means "vapor from rice or millet (food)." Rephrasing this, he comes up with the useful (but somewhat awkward) term "finest matter influences."

Brought into play by a medical practitioner when diagnosing a client, in one of its guises this "finest matter influence" was found within each individual human body. There it was closely related to what other medical systems would term "predisposing" conditions or causes. If one's internal "finest matter influence" was functioning properly, one would be immune to the other, and opposite, aspect of "finest matter influence." This other aspect was a disease-causing force that was carried one's way by the "wind" (*feng*, the word had a complex of meanings).

In Chinese medical thought, "finest matter influence" (*qi*) in its capacity as predisposing cause (within each human) enabled a practitioner to explain why one person came down sick when blown on by an unseasonable "wind" (*feng*), whereas another person who had been blown on by the same *feng* remained perfectly healthy. The first person's *qi* was out of balance and was partially or totally dysfunctional: the second person's *qi* was in standard good condition, and preconditioned him or her not to be susceptible to evil or untimely "winds."

Influences and analogies

Now that we have examined some of the permutations of the categories of Chinese medical thought which, through the application of "human reason," had been brought into being during the late Warring States and early Han periods, we are in a position to mention some of the socio–cultural–political conditions which might have been influential in shaping that thought. Thus for example, when referring to the various parts of the human body, Chinese classical sources often use terms like chief depository, depot, fortress, palace, barrier wall. These terms are obviously analogous to the various military constructions and urban fortifications put up in Han times to stem the violence of localistic feudal magnates.

No less obvious, was the formative influence of followers of the Chinese scholar and reformer, K'ung-fu-tzu, known to Europeans as Confucius (551–479 BCE): Confucius lived during the late Warring States and early Han periods. While he was still alive, few men of consequence listened to what he said. However, as reworked by the scholar Hsun-tzu (fl 238 BCE) and by the principal advisors of the Han Emperor, Wu (156–87 BCE), the Confucian message became, in effect, the official ideology of the Han State. This was a remarkable transformation.

Within the political sphere under the Emperor Wu, the essence of Confucianism was that the ruler and his under officers, both at the center and in the localities, should exemplify the Ideal. Emperors and officials were expected not only to lead exemplary lives, they were also required to antici-pate the future needs and expectations of those they ruled. Taking into account the "correspondence" between macrocosm (in this case the natural environ-ment of the Chinese Empire) and microcosm (the ruler and his under-officers), it was held that under a just ruler who upheld the Ideal, harvests would be plentiful, the empire would be at peace, there would be no devastating floods or epidemics. In short, the Emperor would enjoy the Mandate of Heaven.

Within the medical literature, an essay from the Emperor Wu's period in the *Inner Classic* spoke in analogous, almost identical terms about how a gentleman could preserve himself in good health. In his behavior, the gentleman was always to follow "the mean." He was not to engage to excess in any activity whether at the office, during meals, on the playing fields or while hunting, or in bed with his partner. He was on all occasions to control his emotions, to perform proper rites of obeisance to his ancestors, to remain loyal to his family, friends and so on.

Through this *consciously self-imposed* behavior, according to the Confucian message, the gentleman would keep his internal *qi* in good order. This meant that he would not be predisposed to fall ill from any "disease agent" coming in from the outside, and that he could expect to live a long and healthy life. It will be noticed that there was no mention in any of this of supernatural forces or gods: Confucianism was an ethical system, not a religion. It will also be noticed that it posited a society run by and for males in which women were subordinate beings.

So long as the Han dynasty kept the lid on the chaos which always lay just beneath the surface in China, the Confucian message seemed relevant, both as state policy and as a guide to civil servants' life-style. However, after things fell apart in 220 CE, chaos remained the order of the day for the next 400 years. Not until 618, with the coming into power of the T'ang dynasty, was China again re-united. During the long era of unrest and disorder, the Confucian message temporarily fell into disrepute. In the interval, there was a great stirring of interest in the message of salvation brought in along the southern trade routes from India. The message was that of the Buddha (*c.* 500 BCE).

As we saw in Chapter 5, in India, the role of the Buddha's medico-religious teachings in the making of Ayurvédic medicine is less than clear. But as it emerged in China 800 years later, the Buddha's teachings seemed to offer a war-weary peasantry hope of better things to come in their next reincarnation. And of more immediate relevance to peasants, the monkly inhabitants of flourishing Buddhist monasteries had taken to performing miracle cures in the name of their founder, the "King of Physicians."

Confronted with the increasing popularity of Buddhists sects among the peasantry, the residual Confucian element in what was left of the old Civil Service finally pulled itself together and, after 618 CE, with the coming of the T'ang dynasty, managed to wipe out most of the Buddhists' gains. Monasteries were confiscated, statues of the Buddha were smashed or buried (in hope of better days) and thousands of tax-free monks were forced to return to normal civilian life (as tax-payers).

At the intellectual level, paralleling these political developments, were Chinese medical scholars' vain attempts to incorporate the central tenets of India's Ayurvédic medicine into their own intellectual traditions as set forth in the *Inner Classic*. Attempts at synthesis worked no better with the *Inner Classic*'s temporary replacement, the collection of 81 essays brought together in the late first and early second centuries CE known as the *Classic of Difficult Issues*.

The principal stumbling block Chinese scholars confronted in Ayurvédic medicine was the three *dosas* (or forces). If you review what was said about them in Chapter 5 you will see why: *dosas* were obviously incompatible with Chinese medico-philosophical conceptual patterns. Yet, in all this it is important to realize that an intellectual interchange between Indian medicine and Chinese medicine *was* at least attempted, even though, in the event, it failed.

More important in the actual long-term development of Chinese medicine were the centuries of mutual repulsion followed by centuries of interchange between standard Confucian medicine, the Medicine of Systematic Correspondences, and Taoism.

Founded in the sixth century BCE by a philosopher (Lao-Tse) who preached "the Way" (Tao), Taoism was originally a return-to-nature cult. This held that mental and physical good health were only to be achieved by living in rural isolation in harmony with nature. Standing openly at odds with the urbane, sophisticated behavioral code upheld by the followers of Confucius and their mandarin clientele, early Taoists did what came naturally. They were not afraid to work with their hands and to mix with the peasantry. In time, some scholars found Taoist doctrines to be persuasive and, in the process of making them their own, rubbed off some doctrinal rough edges. We now know that a few Taoist treatises on medicine were among the several hundred included in the *Inner Classic of the Yellow Sovereign* in the form it had achieved by 260 BCE.

Yet, during the Han period and in the 700 years that followed (until the twelfth century CE) Taoist theorists stood well clear of most of the concepts central to the Medicine of Systematic Correspondences (which, as we have seen, was the centerpiece of classical Chinese medicine). However, there was one important exception: in this area *yin-yang* concepts came into play.

During their first millennium, Taoists accepted one of the several *yin-yang* principles to the exclusion of all others. The chosen concept held that the female of the species represented the *yin* principle. This necessarily had to complement the *yang* principle found in every male and, more particularly, in every male's semen. According to Taoist teaching, to enjoy a healthy adult life and a sensuous old age, a man had to build up his supply of semen and keep it flowing. By so doing, he would encourage "process" (the essence of life) and delay stagnation.

In preparation for this, adolescent males were encouraged to masturbate daily. Moving forward in the stages of human existence, Taoists prescribed that adult males have sexual intercourse with many women. Combining in the course of this activity two aspects of "process," they were to delay coming to climax so that they would be able to absorb large quantities of the woman's *yin* when she climaxed. Then, after mutual delivery had been made, the man's body rushed to produce more semen: its production was the second element of "process." All this was described in further detail in the late eighteenth century by Cao Tingdon (1699–1785), a medical writer who apparently practiced what he preached and lived to the age of 86.

Going beyond sexual therapy (seen as a preventive of the degenerative processes of old age), Taoist practitioners in the first millennium CE also made very considerable use of drugs (*yao*) for preventive and for curative purposes. In the absence of modern understandings derived from chemistry (in the West, a 1790s' creation which in any case might not even at that time have been of any interest to them), Taoists thought in terms of categories of properties. One of the most important of a drug's properties was its "taste." A drug which was sour or bitter or sweet was seen as an appropriate cure for diseases in category "x" or "y." Disease categories themselves were established along a range of fever or non-fever states.

Based solidly as they were on elite Chinese conceptual sets, during the first millennium Taoists and other practitioners who used drugs for curative purposes compiled an impressive number of case studies. However, no one during these 1,000 years thought to critically appraise and compare actual results, which might have been rather different from initial "perceptions" about what results should have been.

Then in the twelfth and thirteenth centuries CE, drug scholarship – which, until that time, stood outside the intellectual mainstream – was incorporated fully into the Medicine of Systematic Correspondences. This long-delayed meeting of minds meant that in prescribing a drug, practitioners could now draw on a fuller range of *yin-yang* concepts. In addition to "flavor," drugs were now categorized by their color, with each organ of the patient's body (the microcosm) being associated with one particular color. In keeping with tradition, the relevant parts of the natural environment (the macrocosm) were also associated with a particular color. With the assimilation of Taoist drug knowledge to the Medicine of Systematic Correspondences – twelfth, thirteenth centuries – the range of appropriate treatments was also greatly enlarged. Coming in from distant parts of the Empire and from India and the Spice Islands on giant four-masted Chinese ships (themselves marvels of naval technology which sailed in the other direction all the way to the Red Sea) was a cornucopia of drugs, said to number more than 1,000 in number.

It was also at this time that acupuncture seems to have become *somewhat* more common as one of the curative techniques. To be properly administered, acupuncture required extensive knowledge of one or more of the *yin-yang* systems (no one system was good for all patients) and of one or more of the conceptualizations of where the "conduits" of the human body lay, and with what bodily organ they were in correspondence. However, at no time in the history of Chinese medicine (before the mid-twentieth century) was acupuncture anything more than an auxiliary form of treatment, one technique among many. Very often it was accompanied by the process known as moxibustion: burning bits of fabric on appropriate areas of the skin.

This brings us up to the thirteenth century CE (and beyond) and to a physician's diagnosis of what it was that caused a patient to feel "sick." Once the appropriate knowledge was at hand (in part this was gained by taking a patient's *mai* (pulse) on the *yin* side or the *yang* side and feeling whether it was firm and hard or weak and soft), the practitioner would work out the correspondence between macrocosm and microcosm. For example "winds" (*feng*) blowing from the north-east during the fall of the year under a waning moon were associated with color "x" or "y." This corresponded with human organ "x" or "y," either on the left side or the right. Something, thus, would have to be done to correct the imbalance associated with that "organ."

This level of knowledge would in fact be known to most educated heads of household so, strictly speaking, they didn't need to consult a physician to tell them what they already felt they knew. Meetings between household head and consultant physician might thus result in a no-holds-barred arguing match.

But in "traditional" China, patients whose illnesses were in part brought on by mental stress realized that they might benefit from being able to tell a practicing physician, an *outsider*, how they felt, and then observing how he sorted through relevant categories to arrive at a correspondence which would indicate what sort of curative regime they should undertake. For most people of quality in this situation, more important than the actual treatment, was the outsider physician's careful attention to their psychic needs.

In China before 1840 (where this chapter ends) many moderately well-off city dwellers' illnesses (which they felt they could do nothing about on their own) were probably related to pent up frustrations. Characteristic of their culture was a sense of shame. For example, young adults were ashamed to admit even to themselves that they resented being told what to do by their parents or by aged uncles and grand-parents. They felt caught up in a double bind. On the one hand, their culture taught that filial respect and obedience was obligatory, yet on the other, they felt sick and chronically run down.

Turning in desperation to an *outside* physician, with his deep knowledge of the Medicine of Systematic Correspondences, they finally found they were in the hands of someone they could trust and who understood their problems. Here then, the triangle of curing was complete: the saintly curer (which in secular China, meant the wise and knowledgeable non-family-member physician with his deep knowledge of correspondences); the patient (with his sense of shame brought on by pressures within the family); and the disease, in part or wholly psychosomatic.

And, as of 1840, out in the countryside, triangles of curing were also found, though in detail they were somewhat different. Here, the curer was probably an illiterate wise man or wise women who knew that diseases of the gut or other vital organs were caused by evil forces which had invaded the patient. After taking counsel with the patient, the curer might recommend that he or she burn a wooden comb of the sort used to rid the hair of lice. Putting the ashes of the burnt comb in water, the mixture was then swallowed, on the assumption that the "comb" would rake away the problems in the stomach. An alternative form of sympathetic magic would be to burn an amulet which had been especially created to prevent specific disease "x." Mixed with water, and swallowed, the patient expected that the disease would recognize its error and quickly leave the body.

Conclusion

Within China, on the eve of the Opium Wars with Great Britain which we now know marked the beginning of the end of "traditional China" there were in operation a great diversity of medical systems. Many of those which served the rich and most of those that served the poor provided the necessary elements in the triangle of curing. Though none of these systems were able to confront and overcome serious epidemic disease, as of 1840 neither did any of the medical systems found in the increasingly aggressive and arrogant West.

Further reading

The most coherent general introduction to the history of medicine in China remains that of Paul U. Unschuld (translated in part from the German by Susan Mango and Charles Leslie), *Medicine in China: a history of ideas* (Berkeley: University of California Press, 1985). For a brief trustworthy account of Chinese medicine before it was commercialized for consumption in the West, at the cost of its true identity: Francesca Bray, "Chinese Health Beliefs," in John Hinnells and Royal Porter (eds) *Religion, Health and Suffering* (London: Kegan Paul International, 1999), 187–211.

Chapter 7

The globalization of disease after 1450

Introduction

Thus far we have been examining medical systems developed in the context of a particular cultural grouping: ancient Greek, ancient Chinese and so on. From another perspective, it can be said that each of these medical systems was created by men who believed that the disease situations they themselves confronted were characteristic of their own particular society. Conversely, they believed that neighboring societies, living in a different type of setting, might have their own special diseases. These ideas about the cultural specificity of disease types (who was susceptible to which disease) unfortunately survived long after the breakdown of the physical barriers to permanent, sustained contact between peoples of widely different cultural backgrounds. This breakdown occurred soon after 1450 CE.

As we know, the conquest of the physical space, which before 1450 had separated Old World EurAsian and African civilizations from the New World, was achieved by Europeans using seaworthy ships of a sort they had only recently begun to build. However, we also now know that, by the early fifteenth century, the Chinese, the Indians and some Muslim North African peoples were also building seaworthy ships. Yet, in the event, none of the latter peoples chose to use their fine ships to cross the Atlantic or the Pacific (as the case may be) to the New World.

It would be of huge world historical significance that the discovery/re-discovery and exploitation of the New World (begun in 1492) was achieved by Europeans rather than by some other cultural grouping. As Chinese scholars such as R. Bin Wong have recently pointed out, in and after the mid-fifteenth century, the practice of combining trading/mercantile activities with state-supported conquest and armed violence seems to have become a distinguishing characteristic of the Europeans.

The American continents: a special case

As late as the early months of 1492, the two American continents (North America and South America) contained perhaps a fifth or a sixth of all humankind. Then, in mid-October of that year, disaster struck. From that time onwards, within 20 or 30 years of a "first contact" experience with Europeans in any given setting, the Native Americans left remaining at that setting seldom numbered more than one-tenth of those who had been there before.

Given the vastness of the two continents, "first contact" was not a once-only affair. In the case of South America, "first contact" incidents began in the late 1490s when Spaniards began to trickle over to the mainland from their bases on the Caribbean Islands. Yet, in some parts of the rain forests of Brazil, "first contact" incidents were still taking place 500 years later. For indigenous peoples in the 1990s, these incidents had the same dire consequences as did all those dating from the years immediately after 12 October 1492. With respect to the earlier history of North America, as far as can be determined, the Norse settlers and explorers who were in Newfoundland and the Great Lakes region in the 1360s did not leave behind any long-term contagious diseases.

But in North America, *after* 1492, "first contact" incidents became part of an ongoing process which, on that huge continent, took nearly 300 years to work their way through. Thus, in remote areas such as present-day Oregon, Washington State and the Dakotas, first contact and accompanying population collapse did not happen until after the end of the American Revolutionary War against Britain (1783). This was 300 years after the initial first contact experience in Hispaniola.

That famous/infamous series of incidents began with the landing of Christopher Columbus on the island on 12 October 1492. Within a few decades, the ethnic group he and his crew had first encountered – the Taino – thought to have once been more than one million strong, had almost completely disappeared. Much of what happened during those terrible years remains shrouded in mystery, yet it seems quite certain that most Taino were victims of newly imported diseases and of a policy which purposefully destroyed an entire people and its cultural artifacts. Some aspects of this policy were graphically described by Bartholomé de Las Casas, a Dominican friar who came to Hispaniola in 1502. In his reports back to Spain, Las Casas created what was called the "Black Legend."

Similarly, in coastal North America, beginning in 1622 in the Virginia Colony (founded in 1607) and in 1637 in Massachusetts (founded in 1620), English settlers began to systematically destroy indigenous peoples. Though at times they regarded Native Americans as necessary allies against the French, as soon as the latter were defeated and expelled (with the fall of Quebec City in 1759 and then with the Peace of Paris in 1763), English and other European immigrant settlers had no qualms about killing off all Native Americans who stood in their way. Similarly, in Australia and the Island Pacific, a half century after first contact with whites (effectively beginning in the time of Captain James Cook in the 1780s), indigenous populations had been brought to the brink of extinction.

It is now understood that the massive reduction in the number of Native American and Island Pacific peoples – one-tenth what it had been before contact – was caused by a combination of three factors: (1) the actual diseases the invaders brought with them; (2) the settlers' genocidal practices – of the sort described by Las Casas – and, in the face of these horrible happenings; (3) the collapse of indigenous societies themselves. Their life-worlds shattered, and their triangles of curing wrecked, Native Americans and Pacific islanders failed to reproduce or to keep their newborn infants alive.

Explanations: Old World disease patterns and mind-sets

By 1450 almost the whole of the Old World (EurAsia and coastal North Africa) was well along in the process of becoming a unified disease zone. Long before that date, sophisticated Arab and Indian and Chinese businessmen and traders were crossing and re-crossing the Arabian Sea, the Indian Ocean and the South China Sea in large well-manned ships to visit focal points of progressive enterprise. In terms of global trade, western Europe was marginal. However, local peddlers, touring scholars, missionaries, mercenary soldiers and other agents did manage to maintain enough links with the Middle East to keep western Europe within the larger EurAsian disease zone.

Then, beginning around 1450, breaking out of the impoverished homeland that jutted out into the Atlantic, the Portuguese began to force their way into the Asians' and Arabs' trading networks. They first attacked coastal North Africa, then sailed around to the West African bulge, then round the Cape and northward along the coast to East Africa. From there, working their way further eastward on heavily armored ships with which they shelled and destroyed everybody else's shipping, the Portuguese proceeded to India (Goa) and finally on to China (Macao). Not to be outdone by their tiny neighbor, in 1492, the Catholic monarch of Castile (Isabella) with the support of her husband, Ferdinand, King of Aragon, invested in the expedition (headed by Columbus) which attempted to reach China and its fabled treasures by sailing west, rather than east as the Portuguese were doing.

Recent detailed studies have shown that most of the western European laymen who joined the fleets going out to the New World in and after 1492 were men-on-the-make. (In saying this I have purposefully excluded priests, monks and women: in early years, the latter were few in number). At home in Europe, none of these men-on-the-make had managed to achieve what Old World societies regarded as high status, either because of accidents of birth (aristocrats and gentlemen were "born" not made), or because they had failed to contract an advantageous marriage, or because they had failed in business dealing, or because of general bad luck. Leaving European ports with the expectation that their future lay in their own hands, these rugged

men-on-the-make assumed that if they managed to survive the rigors of
the unknown places beyond the seas and became wealthy, they would return
to their natal lands and buy their way (or at least their children's way) into
high status.

In short, these western Europeans were opportunists who – after escaping
the moral bonds imposed by their home communities – were prepared to
do *anything* to further their personal goals. Added to these characteristics,
were the special traits of the Iberians (denizens of the Spanish kingdoms
and of Portugal) who claimed to be descended from the Gothic peoples
who had come into the land in the late Roman period. With the exiling
of the Jews from the Spanish lands in 1492, and the fall of Granada and
the murder of all remaining Muslims in the same year, employment opportunities at home for mercenary soldiers and for hireling thugs melted away.
Accepting this reality, many of them made their way to the New World
to seek their fortune.

Development and disease

The literate few Iberians and Italians who sailed to America in the fifteenth,
sixteenth and seventeenth centuries had a rough idea about what Hippocrates
(in "Airs, Waters, Places") and later medico-philosophical synthesizers had
said about disease causation. These approved writers held that someone
might come down sick with a serious illness if he or she had recently undergone a "change" of climate or other dramatic alterations in life-style.

If the Hippocratic paradigm were correct, it should have been Columbus
and later European adventurers who came down sick with fatal diseases
after they left their home environment. Yet, in the event, it was the pagan
New World peoples they met and mixed with who, in very large numbers,
fell sick and died of diseases that seemed to leave the Europeans untouched.

As is well known, within a few years of their first arrival, Iberian Europeans
began to realize that, in addition to mining silver, gold and other precious
minerals for export back to the Catholic Kings in Spain, it was necessary to
plant and harvest crops and to raise cattle and the like in order to supplement the foodstuffs brought in so irregularly from the Old World. They also
finally realized that indigenous New World peoples tended to die off if made
to work as slaves on European enterprises. Accordingly, in order to further
their projects, the Europeans cast around for an alternative labor supply.

As it happened, by the early 1500s the Portuguese, the Iberian neighbors
of the Spanish, were in the process of establishing large slave depots on the
central west African coast (now Angola). Despite initial protests from their
respective home governments, out in the colonies, Portuguese slave ship
agents and Spanish slave purchasers very soon established a *modus vivendi*.
With it, the infamous transatlantic slave trade came into existence. A few
decades later, with the eclipse of Portuguese enterprise, first Dutch, and

then English and Scottish slave ship owners provided the transport needed to bring more than 15,000,000 African slaves to the New World. Funding was provided by venture capitalists in Antwerp, London, Amsterdam, Augsburg and (between 1557 and 1627) Genoa.

With this, a working prototype of all later development projects came into being. At the center of the world-encompassing web of enterprise were venture capitalists, based in a handful of great European cities, who funded enterprises intended to bring in a huge return on investment. The enterprises were usually of the sort that collected or grew Non-western raw materials which would then be shipped to western Europe.

In the case of the Americas, by the early sixteenth century Europe's venture capitalists were funding the ships which brought fine manufactured cotton cloth from India to coastal Africa where it was handed over to local African leaders in exchange for slaves abducted from neighboring African societies. These slaves were then shipped across the Atlantic to provide the labor force needed on New World development projects.

One of the early types of development consisted of the sugar cane plantations of coastal Brazil and the Caribbean Islands. Grown and initially processed in the New World, when shipped across the Atlantic and further refined, cane sugar created an entirely new form of consumer demand. Because of its novelty and its popularity among ordinary people who had never before spent money on such trivialities, cane sugar did much to establish the pattern for our modern consumer society.

Setting the tone for later consumer societies, sixteenth-century European venture capitalists at the center of the worldwide web did not allow themselves to be swayed by moral concerns. They themselves were gentlemen. This meant that they could regard everyone else in the enterprise – ship crews, slaves, factors (merchants' traders) and plantation managers in the New World or in the far Pacific – as low status people who could be used for any purpose, whatever the consequences. In short, gentleman venture capitalists regarded the lives of their "factors" and servants as expendable.

Exemplifying this attitude, in the case of fellow white men in the far Pacific, were the practices of the Netherlands' East India Company (established in 1602). With its headquarters in Amsterdam and its "factories" (trading bases) in Indonesia, the Company could not fail to be aware of the short life-expectancies of its "factors" and servants out in the far Pacific. Indeed, in the 200 years after 1602, early death from fevers, dysentery and other water-related diseases found in the Archipelago drained away the lives of huge numbers of young men who otherwise would have remained at home and contributed to population growth in the Netherlands. As it was, between 1662 and 1795, Dutch population size remained static. Here then, by tending to "business" and not worrying about moral issues, the great merchant families of Amsterdam were able to build up and retain hegemonic control over Dutch society.

Disease imports to the Non-west

In the first decades of exchange between the Old World and the Americas, the principal lethal diseases appear to have been influenza, smallpox, measles, typhus and malaria. With the establishment of the slave trade directly between west African ports and Brazil and the West Indies, and the return trade from the Americas to western Europe and thence south along the West African coast, the creation of a unified transatlantic disease zone was finally complete. Now, in addition to the diseases of western Europe and Asia, the New World was also subjected to a full range of African illnesses. Some of these, for example *falciparum* malaria, were far more lethal than the earlier malarial form (*vivax* malaria) which some scholars hold had been brought in to coastal North America from marshlands in western Europe.

Complicating matters, each killer disease actually consisted of two or more variant types. In the case of smallpox, there were three main variants, *Variola major*, *Variola minor*, *Variola intermedius*. When examined in sophisticated laboratories in the early 1970s, there were found to be a total of 450 sub-strains of smallpox, eight of them *Variola major*.

Each disease had its own specific causal agent (pathogen) and its own specific means of transmission. Some, as in the case of smallpox, needed no non-human intermediary. That virus was transmitted directly from one human to another, either through breathing air exhaled by a victim, or by coming into contact with the scabs or flesh which had dropped off the victim's body, or by coming into contact with a victim's clothing or blankets even weeks after the person had died. Measles, in its variant forms, was also transmitted directly from one infected individual to another.

Another early disease import to the New World was malaria (caused by a *plasmodia*) which was transmitted through an intermediary host, one or another type of mosquito. The malaria *plasmodia* (in one of its three forms) reached its full maturity within the human host, and infected this host's bloodstream, from whence it was transferred to another human, by way of a female mosquito of the appropriate sort (in which the *plasmodia* egg first hatched). Thus, even though the appropriate mosquito types might have been in the New World before the arrival of Columbus, they would only become bearers of malaria when females of their type bit and ingested some of the blood of a malaria-bearing migrant from the Old World. In a somewhat similar way, typhus (its causal agent is the *Rickettsia prowazeki*) was also transmitted to humans via an intermediary host, a human body louse, or to be more precise, the fecal matter deposited on human skin by a body louse.

As of the late fifteenth century, influenza (one of the five principal infectious disease killers newly introduced into the New World) was directly tied to the presence of domesticated animals of the sort not found in the Americas before. Indeed, within weeks of the landing on Hispaniola of Christopher Columbus and his henchmen, with their swine, cattle and other fresh meat on the hoof, local Taino people (until then a million in number) were struck down by swine fever, a form of influenza. Not until December 1518 were the Taino who had survived this epidemic attacked by virulent smallpox.

Thereafter, smallpox seems to have replaced influenza as the New World's principal killing disease. In a parallel development in the far Pacific, beginning in the 1750s, smallpox left by fishermen, indigenous to the island of Timor, who had dried their nets and gear on the north-eastern coast of Australia, became the principal killing disease of that continent's Aboriginal population.

Though only one of the five principal killer diseases brought to the western hemisphere around 1500 was directly linked with mammals (influenza, from swine), it would appear that in the distant past, three of the others (malaria, smallpox and measles) had also been linked in one way or another with EurAsian and African humankind's animal companions. As we saw in Chapter 1, in the era between *c.* 13,000 BCE and early October 1492 CE there were no large mammals in the New World that could be domesticated and brought to live in close proximity to humans. Without close contact with friendly, cuddly animals of this sort, the processes of disease evolution which had occurred in the Old World in pre-historic times after sizeable cities had been established could not take place in the New.

In the case of smallpox (in the forms in which it was last known to ordinary scientists in 1977), the protective material originally used for vaccination against the illness, by Jenner in 1796, was derived from the udder of a cow suffering from cowpox. It would thus seem that through the mutative processes of natural selection, the causal agents of cowpox and smallpox had at some past time hived off from one another, to become two distinct diseases. As of 1977 (when it was abolished in the natural world), smallpox had no non-human host.

Turning again to malaria, African and Asian farmers have recently reminded visiting medical scientists that mosquitoes much prefer the blood of cattle to that of humans; if the two mammal types are in the same barn, the mosquitoes will light on the cattle every time. Thus it is likely that ancestral malaria, probably as found along the banks of the Indus River in India, began as a disease associated with cattle and only later became associated with humans.

Posited as happening at some time on the Indian subcontinent, a similar transference may also have taken place in West Africa where, after 1000 BCE, the cattle-keeping ancestors of today's Fulani mingled on a seasonal basis with agriculturalists. However, among adult Africans who in their lifetime did not travel far from their natal village, malaria would not be much of a problem, given that they had acquired immunity to the local variant while they were young children. Difficulties only began when large numbers of Africans were enslaved and taken far from their natal villages into new malaria zones where the immunity they had acquired to their local variant was not effective against the strange new types to which they were being exposed.

In Europe, by the early 1500s, when black African slavery had already become common in Portuguese ports and elsewhere in that mosquito-pestered little country, virulent malaria had become well established, brought in by the slaves and by their Portuguese captors. Virulent malaria was also well established in the mosquito-pestered flat lands south of Rome where absentee-owner estates held black Africans in bondage. In time, some of these estates became unfit for human habitation and fell derelict.

Acquired immunity

In the half century after 1521 (when smallpox first struck the Aztec metropolis, Tenochtitlán), one reason why first generation white immigrants were convinced that they were chosen by God to inherit the western hemisphere was that they seemed to be immune to the sickness which was causing such havoc among indigenous populations. Medical historians now realize that early sixteenth-century white immunity existed not through the intervention of a supernatural force, but because very mild forms of smallpox were endemic in Europe at the time.

As I hinted earlier, endemic viral infectious diseases, such as smallpox (and yellow fever), tended to light on babies and young children, and rather than killing them all off (thus, in the long term, obliterating the virus's necessary hosts) caused only mild discomfort. In exchange for hosting it, the virus then provided recipients with life-long immunity to all further attacks. In the random logic of natural selection this meant that the infant human host (having served its purpose) would then reach maturity and produce infants, who in turn would host the smallpox virus (or the yellow fever virus) and thus enable it to perpetuate itself.

Like smallpox, a case of measles in one or another of its forms (also caused by a virus), similarly provided life-long immunity or near immunity. From the thirteenth century onwards measles was endemic in Europe, the Middle East and China, though in forms that were slightly different from those known today. Given what we know about its behavior in the 1530s, in EurAsia measles could sustain itself in mild form in interacting village communities numbering only a few thousand people.

Thus it happened that most of the Spanish and other Europeans who happened to be in the once heavily populated Valley of Mexico when measles struck in virulent epidemic form in 1531, found that they personally were immune (or suffered only light cases from which they easily recovered), even though indigenous people all around them were dying in great numbers. This confirmed the Europeans in their belief that Native Americans were cursed by God and that He intended that they should disappear.

In common with measles and smallpox, a mild attack of typhus also conferred life-time near-immunity to the disease. At a time when Spaniards abhorred bathing or changing their underclothes, it is likely that most of them were infested with body lice and that since infancy they had had experience with mild forms of typhus. By way of contrast, Native Americans abhorred body filth and bathed as frequently as circumstances permitted. Unfortunately, in prejudiced Spanish minds, this custom linked the peoples of the New World (none of whom had ever heard of the Prophet Muhammad or of Christ) with the ritually-well-washed Muslims who – until they had been killed off or sent into exile by Queen Isabella in 1492 – had inhabited Andalusia in southern Spain.

Disease and the destruction of New World populations

Within 30 or 40 years of "first contact" (beginning in October 1492) in any particular "disease region" in the New World indigenous population numbers dropped precipitously, generally leaving only one person alive where there had been ten before. In defining a "disease region" one must take into account the special characteristics of the disease involved.

In the case of measles (which ravaged the Valley of Mexico in 1531–32) the "disease region" would be relatively small and self-contained, since the disease is highly contagious, usually acquired through direct contact with a sick person or with virus-laden droplets in the air which had been expelled from the lungs of the sick one. Here, the time between infection and the appearance of symptoms (the incubation period) was brief, limiting the geographic scope of disease transmission.

But the situation was quite different in the case of smallpox. Here, the virus causal agent was present in a bearer for a week or more before the person came down sick. During that time a Native American who happened to be in the business of carrying news and trade-goods between distant places might be able to travel 50 or 60 kilometers a day. This meant he might have traveled three or four hundred kilometers from the epicenter of a smallpox epidemic before falling sick and becoming an infective agent. For this reason, the "disease region" of smallpox might well include whole territories that had not yet been visited by whites.

The most famous example is that of the Incas of Peru, until the mid-1520s, rulers of a mighty empire that stretched for hundreds of kilometers along the Andes and the west coast of South America. Smallpox, probably brought in by Native American runners from the north, ravaged the heart of the empire in 1524–25. This was six years before the arrival of man-on-the-make Francisco Pizarro in 1531. In its early stages the epidemic killed the Inca king and many of the royal family, leading to a disputed succession and civil war. In the midst of this, Conquistador Pizarro (himself immune to smallpox) had no difficulty in coming in and taking charge.

We have already answered *part* of the rhetorical question, "Why did they die?". As we have pointed out, until 1492 no New World person had ever come into contact with smallpox or any other of Europe's cornucopia of infectious diseases. Not having acquired any immunity to these diseases, when they struck, New World peoples died in terrifyingly large numbers.

Yet, there may well be more to it than that. As every veterinarian (animal doctor) knows, no matter what disease hits a herd of cattle, some beasts survive, exemplifying the principle of "herd immunity." Of course, when dealing with domesticated animals it is assumed that a human owner is on hand to feed and water the sick animals until they recover. In the case of human beings, similar requirements have to be met.

Thus, wherever in the Old World smallpox broke out in lethal form, there would always be some responsible older people around (who had acquired immunity as children) to serve as carers during the ten to 12 days a small-pox patient was semi-delirious and unable to manage for her- or himself. But in the Americas, when an epidemic of smallpox first broke out as in the Valley of Mexico in 1520 or in the Pequot lands of New England in 1634, there would be no indigenous people around who had acquired immunity. Any family member brave enough to bring water and food to a sick person would soon fall sick herself. This sort of happening didn't have to repeat itself very often before all sane persons took to their heels and fled, spreading contagion into the countryside as they ran along. A famous example was the epidemic crisis that hit the Andean city of Arequipa and its densely populated hinterland in 1589, leaving more than a million dead.

Living as we do more than four hundred years after these terrible events, and in the absence of specimens of the disease casual agents that wrought such havoc (which could be analyzed using modern laboratory techniques), we can do no more than speculate about what happened and why.

This brings us to contentious topics. The first involves assessing the genetic make up of (long dead) individuals in particular population groups. The second is to assess the degree of disease-resistance *diversity* that might have been found in any given (long dead) population, say, "Population A" compared to some other (long dead) population, "Population B."

Let me begin with "Population A," the inhabitants of western Europe around 1200 CE. It is now known that the ancestors of the people who had come to settle in western Europe before 1200 CE had moved there from many far off regions. Some of these ancestors (or ancestral groupings) had come from central and western Asia, some from the Middle East and North Africa, some from eastern Europe and so on. Each of these ancestral group-ings had their own distinctive genetic inheritance and, with it, their own distinctive clustering of chromosomes. At the level of the individual, each chromosome carried disease resistance units known as *alleles*.

After each of these various ancestors (ancestral groupings) settled down in western Europe, they and their progeny intermarried with women and men descended from other ancestral groupings. Happening over the course of several thousand years, emerging out of this mixing process were late-medieval Europeans. They were very much a mongrel people.

Because of this complex genetic situation in western Europe, there were a large number of possible combinations of alleles (disease resistance units) in the late medieval population. Indeed, given that alleles are attached to chromosomes, and that brothers and sisters do not share the same chromosomes, even siblings had slightly different immune systems. Next door neighbors also carried combinations that differed one from the other.

Thus, a disease pathogen attacking any member of the allele-rich population that was western Europe in the years after 1450 (the date after which most immigrants to the New World were born) would, in assaulting each individual person, confront a slightly different immune system. Sorting out these differences in defense systems and overcoming them one by one presumably had the potential to slow down the movement of the disease. It might even encourage it to remain in mild endemic form, rather than breaking out as a virulent epidemic. This then (in simplified form) was the situation in western Europe.

But in the New World, the accidents of settlement history were entirely different. Though much of this remains conjectural, it would seem that as of 11 October 1492 (the eve of Columbus' landing) the entire population of the Americas was descended from only four or five small Asian groupings (each perhaps under a dominant Patriarch). At various times 12 or 13 thousand years ago these small groups (two or three hundred strong) had made their way across dry land between present day Siberia and Alaska. Some of the descendants of these groups gradually made their way southwards, eventually to southern Chile.

Because the number of founding ancestors was very small (perhaps only a few dominant Patriarchs had initially been involved in the migration), the number of alleles possessed by their millions of descendants several thousand years later was also small when compared to mixed-breed European populations (with their far-flung and varied ancestral roots). It can be argued that as a result, in the whole of New World there was not much diversity in alleles. This meant that an epidemic disease, such as measles or smallpox, at work in that population, had far fewer immune system differences to overcome than would have been the case in western Europe. This would perhaps explain why, in the Valley of Mexico, measles went berserk every 20 or 30 years. Measles hit the Valley in epidemic form in 1531–32, in 1563–64, in 1592–93, and in 1595–97, leaving tens of thousands of people dead, many of them children.

Records kept in New Spain by Catholic priests suggest that later epidemics were marginally less severe. Perhaps this was because Spanish settler males (in the absence of Spanish females) tended to sleep around with Native American women and, in the process, gradually enriched the local gene bank and, with it, the diversity of alleles found in the population. Yet the lessening severity of epidemics in places that had been repeatedly ravished early on – such as the Valley of Mexico – may also be related to gradual mutations in the viral disease agents themselves.

Using the slippery technique, "argument by analogy" we can remind ourselves that a disease not before known in mainland Europe – venereal syphilis – had also been highly virulent when it first appeared in 1494 among military men and prostitutes in Italy and France. According to alarmists' reports at the time, heralding their early death, within a few weeks of contracting the disease the noses and penises of syphilis victims dropped off. However, 50 years later, medical authorities claimed that venereal syphilis had lost some of its most alarming symptoms and now took many years to complete its lethal work. If this were true, it would suggest that the disease had adjusted itself to a new environment, taking care not to kill off victims before they had time to breed children who could later serve as disease hosts.

A somewhat similar mutation in disease behavior (at first highly virulent, then much less so) *may* have happened to the viral agents of smallpox and measles in New Spain after 1650. However, without samples of actual disease causal agents from before and after 1650 that can be tested using modern laboratory techniques, suppositions about such changes remain only that.

Solid arguments, derived from biology, supplement, and may ultimately supersede, earlier "cultural" arguments. One "cultural" argument, most often applied to North America (based on two or three observations by bemused whites), held that according to native custom, whenever a community member fell sick, it was the duty of the whole community to visit, frequently. If the sick person had come down with an air-borne communicable disease – measles or smallpox – the visiting process would obviously put the entire community at risk.

A much less valid, but frequently repeated "cultural" argument, holds that Native Americans, when confronted with smallpox and its sores and pustules commonly resorted to steam baths in search of cleansing and cure. Modern historians who claim that this was the worst thing they could have done, are, unknown to themselves, simply reiterating sixteenth-century Spanish claims that bathing was "evil" – because it was a Muslim custom.

As we have seen throughout this book, "disease" is a reality (synonymous with disease agent/pathogen), but "illness" is – at least in part – a perceptual state. "Illness" (as perceived by "self") can be caused by *individual* misfortune and circumstances. But a state of mind conducive to serious illness would also be found among an entire ethnic group (or, as in the Aztec Empire, a collection of ethnic groups) whose lived-world had totally collapsed.

In the Spanish-ruled lands of America after 1492/1521, native people found themselves in a situation where their heads of government had been killed off by disease or murdered, where all their religious and cultural writings had been burnt, where their cities, temples and aqueducts had been dismantled and destroyed, where their lands had been stolen and their livelihoods destroyed, and where they had all been reduced to the dank equal status of serfs.

Here then, life-worlds of the sort known before the Conquest (not that these had been Gardens of Eden) were replaced by a new life-world in which control of "self" and overall control of the ethnic group were in the hands of an "Other." This "Other" consisted of Spanish landowners, Spanish entrepreneurs, Spanish priests (who insisted in collecting scattered rural communities into tight-packed, disease-ridden "congregations") and – at the center of the development web in Genoa and in northern European cities – gentleman venture capitalists.

In North America, the cast of characters in the "Other" was slightly different (in the English colonies there were no priests to speak of) but the end result was much the same. After the arrival of local whites as land-thieves, individual natives' sense of self-worth and personal identity was shattered.

Within the Americas – North and South – each ethnic group responded to this situation in their own way. In the Valley of Mexico, according to a survey taken in the 1580s, it would seem that survivors married at a younger age than had been the case before 1521, and had more live births. However, it would also seem that parents – demoralized by the Spanish regime – did little to keep their babies alive; the result was population stagnation, or continued decline. Further to the south, in the Andes, it would seem that a high proportion of married young people did not bother to have children at all. Given that very few Native American migrants were coming in, this too resulted in population decline.

A similar situation seems to have prevailed in much of North America. Here, demoralized Native American males often felt that since there would be no future worth living for, there was no point in marrying. Indeed many of them decided that there was no point in doing anything at all other than drink the whiskey and cheap rum which the white folks made available. In the late eighteenth and nineteenth centuries, drunken tribal chieftains readily agreed to treaties which handed over all tribal lands to white occupation, in perpetuity.

But in earlier centuries, some groups of Native Americans had clearly demonstrated that they would not easily accept being made into landless slaves. For example, in the spring of 1519 Aztec warriors had had no trouble in killing off most of the soldiers brought in by Cortés before they themselves were brought low by something other than western armaments. Two years later, when most Aztec warriors were in the process of dying from smallpox, Cortés had no difficulty in defeating them in battle; but then this was not exactly a fair fight.

Turning to the situation in North America, it is known that during the early years, Native Americans fought long and hard against land-grabbing settlers before they too were brought low by something else. In the absence of that "something else" (lethal European-borne diseases) it can be argued that had the full complement of New World people still been around in 1800 or 1850, they would have outnumbered European settlers by a factor of 50 to one. In the days before Gatling guns, man for man, Native American warriors were fully the equal of warriors of European stock.

The supposition that killing diseases (rather than just superior armaments and leadership) made possible the conquest of the Americas by Europe can, in part, be supported by evidence drawn from another part of the world, New Zealand. When, in the late eighteenth century, land-hungry British settlers came to North Island and South Island they found them occupied by the Maori. These people may well have been beneficiaries of a richer inheritance of alleles than were the indigenous people of Australia or the New World.

The Maori themselves had only come to New Zealand as conquerors around 1200 CE. As a peripatetic Polynesian people, it is possible that they had already had experience with some of the disease types found in East Asia. In any case, it would seem that they were not blitzed by European-borne diseases at first contact to the extent that most other Non-western people were. As a result, the Maori were able to retain their societal cohesion and their ability to defend themselves against European aggressors, sometimes using guns purchased from whites. Beneficiaries of a humanitarian governor, in 1840 the status of the Maori as a permanent element in the New Zealand population was recognized by the Waitangi treaty arrangement (this, at any rate is the reading in the Maori-language version of the treaty). Though they lost considerable ground in the next 90 years, by 1935 they were still very much present and were undergoing a major cultural revival. Their integrity and separate identity still intact, the Maori currently account for 15 percent of the population.

World historical consequences

In the New World, the processes of globalization (which were entirely dependent on development and development agents) could not have worked their way to fruition had not key regions in the two continents first been denuded of their Native American population. This denuding process, as we have seen, was achieved through the interaction of three factors: European-imported diseases, European sadistic behaviors and the collapse of Native Americans' lived-worlds.

In world historical terms, in the long run, the denuded region of most consequence was that lying inland from the Gulf of Mexico. Stretching from West Florida to beyond the Mississippi, in the years after 1815 this vast region became the home of *King Cotton*. Without this African slave-grown cotton (and England's own newly discovered reserves of coal), England's fledgling "industrial revolution" would probably have petered out and Britain would have joined Venice and Flanders/Netherlands as the home of yet another failed attempt at modernization.

But as Kenneth Pomeranz nicely demonstrates in his *The Great Divergence: China, Europe and the making of the modern world* (2000), Britain (rather than China – as late as 1750 China still had many things going for it) *did* achieve full modernization. Building on breakthrough achievements first in cotton, then in steam, after 1850 England's gentleman capitalists created the British world economic system. A century later, this world economic system was inherited by America.

Further reading

For Spanish speakers: Sheldon Watts, *Epidemias y Poder: historia, enfermedad, imperialismo* (Barcelona: Editorial Andres Bello, 2000); in English as *Epidemics and History: disease, power and imperialism* (London: Yale University Press, 1997). The five hundredth anniversary of Columbus in America, 1492–1992, saw the production of many books which re-appraised Spanish achievements in the destruction of the New World. Particularly useful is Noble David Cook, *Born to Die: disease and New World conquest, 1492–1650* (Cambridge: Cambridge University Press, 1998) and David Stannard, *American Holocaust: Columbus and the conquest of the New World* (Oxford: Oxford University Press, 1992). An important article on alleles: Francis Black, "An explanation of high death rates among New World peoples when in contact with Old World diseases," *Perspectives in Biology and Medicine* 37 (2) Winter 1994, 292–307. A key book on the making of the modern world: Kenneth Pomeranz, *The Great Divergence: China, Europe and the making of the modern world economy* (Princeton, NJ: Princeton University Press, 2000): an update is the AHR Forum: "Asia and Europe in the World Economy": *American Historical Review* 107 (2) April 2002, 418–80.

Chapter 8

Medicine and disease in the West, 1050–1840

Introduction

This chapter briefly considers what was distinctive about medicine and the medical profession in western Europe in the 800 years or so before the emergence of the European medical scientists who finally broke through the web of customs inherited from ancient times. For a variety of reasons (the precise nature of which is still in dispute among certain breeds of historians and philosophers), this breakthrough would be very long in coming. Four hundred years after Europeans had brought about the beginnings of radical change in one field of human endeavor (economic globalization beginning soon after 1450), European medical practitioners continued to be caught up in their ancient professional web.

A second new beginning

With the collapse of the Roman Empire in the West in the fifth century CE, formal medicine had ceased to exist in those portions of the old Empire and in western Europe as a whole. Thus the recovery for the West, in the mid-eleventh century, of the Galenic interpretation of ancient Greek medical writings through the intermediacy of Muslim writers and the Christian monk translator, Constantinus Africanus (c.1020–27), was of very considerable importance.

Within a primitivized eleventh-century West which was only just beginning to recover from the collapse of centralized authority and the effects of anarchic localism, the regaining of elements of medicine's Great Tradition (translated from the Arabic to Latin by Constantinus) renewed the idea that theorizing about individual men and women's physical health was a legitimate scholarly concern. It also brought into being the conviction that as far as explanations of "dis-ease" and good health were concerned there existed a single set of true concepts which had been validated by Authority in the Golden Age of Wisdom (which is to say, antiquity). These two concepts continued to underlie and to legitimize scholarly endeavors during the fifteenth-century

Italian Renaissance and the early sixteenth-century "recovery of learning" in northern Europe.

In practice, however, the two concepts, (1) that it was legitimate to theorize, and (2) that *true* knowledge – now lost – had been known in the past), tended to counteract each other. Given that the pursuit of theoretical knowledge about man and the natural world was regarded as a scholarly activity best pursued by university dons who were well grounded in the teachings of the philosopher par excellence (Aristotle, 384–322 BCE), the conceptual world in which theorizing took place was at odds with the real world of everyday medieval and early modern lived experience. Until this Aristotelian conceptual world was finally recognized as inappropriate to the study of actual reality (the world around us), the disparate "facts" emerging from casual experimentation with everyday objects and from empirical observation could not be made to fit into any meaningful whole. This generally meant that these "facts" had to be ignored.

In medicine, in the medieval and early modern and eighteenth-century West, just as in the time of al-Razi in tenth-century Baghdad (see pages 40–4), "empirics" (who dealt with "facts") were ridiculed and held up to scorn by the scholarly profession. As we saw earlier, empirics were unorthodox – often illiterate – practitioners and vendors of cures who, through personal experience with sick people, picked up all sorts of understandings about the relationship between disease and cure. However, not being organized in any way, knowledge gained from personal experience was lost when individual empirics retired or died.

By way of contrast, medical doctors who held degrees from prestigious universities such as Paris, Oxford or Cambridge, had a lot going for them. Given that ready access to scholarship was a visible attribute of power, the presence of a scholar-physician in the Court of a prince or great magnate added further to the luster of the employer. Until the very late eighteenth century (in the German lands) and early nineteenth century (in less intellectualized kingdoms), aristocratic/feudal patronage of traditional Galenic "rational" medicine ensured its continued dominance of the field.

That those in authority did not regard scholarly or any other form of medicine as particularly important in maintaining the health of their social inferiors was, however, demonstrated by the virtual neglect of medical provision in the armies of Napoleon (1793–1815). It continued to be neglected in the armies of the British and French and Russians who fought in the Crimean War (1854–56), in the American armies who fought each other in their Civil War (1861–65), in the British army in the Boer War (1899–1902), and in the British, British Empire and French armies in the First World War (1914–18). During all these conflicts, high-ranking military commanders assumed that the "manliness" of their troops would see them through, and that any soldier who fell sick was a malingerer and shirker. In these wars, deaths from improperly treated wounds and from sickness far out-numbered deaths from enemy bullets, sabre slashes or cannon.

Paradigmatic diseases

To illustrate the ambivalent role played – until the mid-nineteenth century – by those who claimed to possess special knowledge about illness, let us briefly examine western Europe's experiences with three well-known diseases: bubonic plague, leprosy and syphilis. For the sake of comparison, I will make brief mention of instances of these diseases in the Non-west.

As every European school girl and boy knows, western Europe was attacked by what most well-informed scholars assume was bubonic plague in 1347. During the next five years, the Black Death killed perhaps a fifth or a quarter of the population. In European folk memory, this was the greatest disease disaster ever to have struck the continent. Given that the European medical profession was, by then, well established and had medical degree-granting programs at Montpellier in France and at several of the Italian universities, it is legitimate to ask about the nature of the medical response.

First, as far as can be determined, no fourteenth-century western European doctor consulted the chronicles that recorded the last occurrence of a plague of this sort in Europe. "Justinian's Plague" as it was later termed had inter-mittently hit western Europe between 541 CE and the late seventh century (it last appeared in England in 687).

Fourteenth-century doctors' apparent ignorance of this earlier plague disaster may be credited to the fact that (as we saw) there had been no medical doctors in western Europe at that time (the medical Dark Ages). However, medical and other fourteenth-century learned commentators *were* quite willing to draw close parallels between the plague in their own time and the "plague" of 427 BCE which the Greek historian Thucydides (c. 460–400 BCE) had reported in his history of the Peloponnesian War (see page 33). Indeed, some accounts of the impact of the Black Death in for example, Siena (a leading city-state in north Italy), follow Thucydides' description almost word for word, and told about fathers deserting sons, sons deserting fathers, corpses lying about everywhere in deserted streets and so on. Here then, the literary model from antiquity had greater explana-tory value than anything fourteenth-century commentators might have seen with their own eyes.

When it came to explaining what had brought on the fourteenth-century plague, most medical doctors fell back upon the same causal agency as did most other Christians: God had sent it to punish people for their sins. Alternatively, the Christian God had permitted Jewish people to go around poisoning the city wells with the plague. In all this, medical doctors contributed nothing new to enlighten the public about what was going on. And, like most other people who had cash reserves or rich friends, when plague threatened their city, most doctors fled to safe refuge in a gentleman's country estate.

Then, in the 1450s, nearly a century *after* the plague had first hit north Italian cities and had taken to reappearing every four or five years, *town magistrates* (not medical men) hit upon the idea that the disease was *contagious*. According to them, it was spread from person to person and most especially by the poor. This meant that the poor – which is to say two-thirds of an ordinary city population – had to submit to the discipline of confinement for the sick in special pest houses, the closure of town markets, the quarantine of travelers by land and of ships coming in by sea.

For our purposes it is important to notice that the core concept under-lying these draconian measures put into force by city magistrates – the concept of contagion – was completely at odds with the Galenic orthodoxy which medical doctors had learned in their universities. Following ancient teachings, the doctors held that sickness was caused by an imbalance in the humors. It was not caused by an invisible something spread from person to person. Intellectually committed to these Galenic notions (see pages 41–2), medical doctors contributed nothing in their official capacities to understanding the causes of plague or how it could be controlled and prevented. In fact, bubonic plague, being spread by fleas carried on many sorts of rodents – not just rats – is not strictly speaking contagious. It is not spread directly from one human to another in the way that smallpox used to be (it was abolished in 1977), and as syphilis still is, spread.

In the event, in the sixteenth and seventeenth centuries, the establish-ment of efficient quarantine control measures in port cities, of *cordon sanitaire* by armed troops and of information networks to warn of the approach of disease danger was all achieved by those European *civil authorities* who purposely ignored or overrode the objections of medical doctors. By creating and enforcing the Ideology of Order in time of plague, princes consider-ably strengthened their hold over their subject populations. Quarantine procedures coincided with the gradual disappearance of plague from western Europe: it last appeared in 1721.

One hundred and twenty years later, in Egypt, Muhammad ʿAli, the Macedonian pasha who ruled the country in the name of the Ottoman Sultan (from 1805–48), also overruled the strong objections of his French medical advisor, the anti-contagionist, Clot Bey. Well informed about the Ideology of Order, Muhammad ʿAli established the quarantines and *cordon sanitaire* which, in 1844, finally brought an end to the visitations of bubonic plague which, since 1347, had been periodically depleting the population of Egypt.

Returning to the situation in western Europe in the fourteenth century, let us turn to the medical response to leprosy. Most literate Europeans at the time considered this to be a stigmatizing disease which they thought especially common among moral reprobates and sexual degenerates. Drawing on the Jewish book of Leviticus and on accounts of parables taught by a Jewish teacher in Palestine during the time of Tiberius Caesar (14–37 CE), early fourteenth-century Christians also held that Jewish people were particularly prone to leprosy. As it happened, because the Jewish religion held literacy and book learning in high regard, a very sizeable proportion of Europe's medical doctors at that time were Jews.

Be this as it may, whatever his motives, in 1363 Guy de Chauliac (at one time the personal physician to Pope Clement VI) published the results of his research into what ancient authority had identified as *true* (as opposed to metaphorical) leprosy. De Chauliac perhaps realized that many people were being accused of being lepers by vindictive enemies or family members who simply wanted them out of the way.

The standard procedure required that a jury "find" the accused were lepers. Through these legal devices (an accusation before a magistrate, followed by a jury trial), before 1363 numerous inconvenient heirs to estates, female scolds, and Jews whose toes, fingers, noses and nerve endings were still intact (which they would not have been had the accused actually had full-blown leprosy) had been made to disappear behind the walls of leprosariums.

The publication (in manuscript copies) of de Chauliac's guide to the true marks of leprosy in 1363 made the process of banishing an unwanted person to a leprosy prison much more difficult. Jury members who took their duties seriously could now closely examine the suspect's person and compare what they saw with what the new medical guide said were the true symptoms and marks of the disease. Many jurors proved to be honest men. Not by coincidence, soon after 1363 most of Europe's huge number of special purpose prisons for lepers fell vacant for want of inmates. In this way, medical authority (Guy de Chauliac) had successfully rid Europe of what in the years between 1090 and 1363 had been considered to be a major disease threat.

Our third paradigmatic disease is syphilis. In the late 1490s most medical authorities forced themselves to accept that this often lethal venereal disease was entirely new to Europe. This was a painful admission, given that the illness had not been mentioned in any of the writings of Galen or in any of the growing corpus of writings from ancient Greece in the original Greek, which even then were in the process of being recovered from libraries in the Middle East and southern Europe by Renaissance scholars.

We now know that syphilis (*Treponema pallidum* or *Treponema S.*) is closely related to yaws (*Treponema Y*) and to *Treponema M* and *C* and that yaws (a non-venereal disease) was found in the New World in 1492. Our supposition is that Columbus' sailor crews picked up yaws while sexually assaulting Taino women on Hispaniola. The disease then mutated in their bodies on the voyage back to Spain to become the *Treponema pallidum* which suddenly was so much in evidence among the French mercenary army which invaded Italy in 1494.

In any case, drawing on analogies derived from the medical literature of the past, many of Europe's sixteenth-century medical doctors thought to recommend a course of mercury as treatment for syphilis. However, they knew that mercury was a deadly poison, and that its use as treatment would cause all sorts of unpleasant side-effects, including loss of hair and teeth. Accordingly, canny medical doctors tended to recommend that anyone who needed treatment take himself off to a barber or some other unorthodox curer. In that way, should anything go wrong, the medical doctor would not be held responsible, at the cost of his reputation. The arrival of syphilis on the European scene thus much enlarged the number of opportunities available for unorthodox curers.

The opening up of the medical marketplace

Beginning in the 1520s, Paracelsus (1493–1541) the son of an obscure Swiss miner, began to travel around the countryside, consulting earnestly with working people about what they were doing and what they knew about the natural world around them. He became particularly interested in disease forms and in ways to recover good health. Paracelsus concluded that nothing that Galen, the ancient Greeks, or the medical doctors of his day said about these matters made sense.

He also concluded that instead of placing one's faith in the humors, one should place reliance on the chemicals God had provided for human use. Paracelsus was particularly keen on the use of antimony (a poison) as an antidote to diseases which had poisoned the body. This use of a poison to cure a poison ("like curing like") was diametrically opposed to the Galenic idea that a disease condition could best be cured by its opposite.

Though not much known during his lifetime, after his death in 1541, Paracelsus' many writings were published (one of the many triumphs in the early history of the printing press, a Chinese invention re-invented in Mainz, Germany, in the 1450s). By the end of the sixteenth century and during much of the seventeenth century Paracelsus' chemical doctrines were hotly debated in medical schools in France and elsewhere on the continent.

For us, the principal importance of this scholarly interest in Paracelsus is that for the first time in the West, a viable non-folk alternative to Galenic medicine had come into being. Whatever the validity of his doctrines, Paracelsus had broken through the ancient mold in medicine, just as in the 1620s England's Francis Bacon had reputedly broken through the ancient mold in the sciences in general. In his *Instaurati Magna* (the Great Instauration) the corrupt Lord Chancellor had demanded that the authority of Aristotle be recognized as a hindrance to progress in all human endeavors. Bacon had claimed that the betterment of mankind's estate (control over nature, "development") could only be advanced if Aristotle and his kind were locked away in the museum of obsolete ideas. However, 200 years later, Aristotle still remained well entrenched in many university departments.

Yet, in the eighteenth century, in England, the downward spread of prosperity brought in from the colonial exploitation of the Americas (including slave-grown sugar in the West Indies: see page 89) brought with it a great new burst of consumer demand. Through the accidents of history, this demand was able to sustain itself and to increase in volume from one decade to the next. Included in the things demanded by consumers were sure cures for all disease conditions. Given that in 1800 the formal medical profession was no more able to offer effective cures for any disease than it had been in 1100, this meant that the populace increasingly turned to vendors of wonder drugs who promised to cure any condition for a few pence.

The commercialization of demands for medicine, first in England, and then at some remove in France, forcibly reminded the practitioners of formal medicine that unless they shaped up, turned away from Galenic "rational" medicine, and came up with sensible answers to modern medical problems they would become obsolete. Some met this threat by peddling wonder-drugs on the side.

In the event, however, it was the demand by princely patrons and their funding agencies in the German lands (rather than the demands of ordinary consumers in England) which finally led to the creation of what we now regard as modern medicine. The day of the research institute had finally dawned.

Further reading

The best place to begin is the bibliography found in Sheldon Watts, *Epidemics and History: disease, power and imperialism* (London: Yale University Press, 1997).

Chapter 9

The birth of modern scientific medicine

The German lands contrasted with the United Kingdom and the British in India

Introduction

Students in search of the birthplace of modern scientific medicine must necessarily first turn to the German lands in the 30 years before, and the 40 years after, Unification (in 1870–71). There, between 1840 and 1910, for the first time ever, there was a coming together of several distinct strands of thought. These eventually resolved themselves into the single strand which held that *true scientific knowledge* of each specific disease causal agent and its relationship to humankind would, in the not too distant future, bridge the age-old gap between medical theories and effective therapeutic practice.

Though "eventually" had yet to happen in 1910 (the actual therapeutic revolution did not occur until the 1940s – see Chapter 10 – the continuing *faith* that it would happen in the foreseeable future continued to impel German state administrators to provide lavish funding for university-based research laboratories staffed by full-time medical scientists. Accompanying this, beginning in 1869, graduates of state-funded medical schools were provided with opportunities for life-time careers as medical doctors in the employ of state-funded medical insurance schemes for working-men and civil servants. Other talented graduates were given employment as full-time laboratory research scientists.

Here then, both in the universities, and in the German-speaking world as a whole, there was a growing constituency of influential people who shared the faith that massive government investment in medical research was well worthwhile. And though the therapeutic pay-off was delayed, what ultimately made it possible were the breakthroughs made after 1876 in secure, scientifically based knowledge about the causal agents of the particular *infectious* diseases that were responsible for more than half of all deaths in western Europe, in North America and in the colonial world.

The pre-eminent personage in all this was Robert Koch of north Germany (1843–1910), discoverer of the causal agent of anthrax (1876), of tuberculosis (1882), and of cholera (1883–84). In the course of making his revolutionary findings, Koch devised radically new uses for microscopes by preparing pure cultures of pathogen "X" or pathogen "Y" for microscopical examination, new staining techniques and new, improved lenses. Moreover, while formalizing what modern laboratory medical science meant, Koch worked closely with other German medical scientists (such as Paul Ehrlich, discoverer, in 1909, of the first "magic bullet" against venereal syphilis).

In 1884, one of Koch's pupils, (Georg Gaffky, 1850–1918), discovered the causal agent of typhoid, another major urban killer disease. During these years other pupils and scientists using Koch's laboratory methods discovered the causal agents of diphtheria, pneumonia, tetanus, gonorrhea and cerebrospinal meningitis. Koch also worked with young visiting scholars from overseas (most famously, with Shibasaburo Kitasato of Japan – discoverer of the causal agent of bubonic plague) in establishing the global pre-eminence of laboratory science. But this brings us ahead of our story.

In this chapter, I will briefly mention the various strands of thought and the institutional patternings which, in the German lands from the 1790s onwards, formed the contextual background against which the Laboratory Revolution in medicine finally arose. Then, turning to the United Kingdom, I will discuss some of the ways in which its politicians and leading medical establishment figures blocked progress along German lines until the early years of the twentieth century. In Britain there was no state funding for laboratory research until 1913.

Yet, among the clouds overhanging the Imperial islands, there were a few rays of sunshine. As we will see, during the years after 1830, London-based administrators cobbled together a disease prevention technique that proved to be remarkably effective. Misleadingly called sanitary "science," it was based on Greco-Roman understandings of disease causation. But despite its shaky theoretical basis, when given practical application after 1870, modified forms of sanitary science were instrumental in considerably extending the life expectancy of British urban populations.

At the end of the chapter, looking at implications in the Non-west, we will see that a few months before the opening of the Suez Canal, which cut across Egypt, in 1869, the governing elite of Britain introduced a topsy-turvy theory of disease into India. At the same time, they established a financial regime which would not permit the establishment of "sanitary" policies of the sort being applied to such good effect in Britain itself. In addition to causing millions of unnecessary deaths in India in the eight decades after 1868, the result was to burden the subcontinent with medically-unsound ideologies from which it has been difficult for post-independence generations to escape.

The German lands: the intellectual and institutional background

As is well known, until the early 1790s the nation we now know as "Germany" consisted of a multiplicity of small and medium-sized political entities. Then, beginning in 1792 and continuing through the time of Napoleon, the French invaded and subdued the German lands. Later at the Congress of Vienna in 1815, the victorious "allies" (Russia, the UK, the Hapsburg Empire and so on) re-arranged the political map of Europe, leaving a "Germany" which consisted of 38 states and territories.

Unlike the Anglo-Scottish island kingdom, with its ruling elite based on London, and the French polity centered on Paris, until well after Unification in 1871 there was no one dominant city in the German lands. This multi-centeredness meant, among other things, that German rulers did not interest themselves in acquiring overseas empires and in frittering away talent overseas.

Multi-centeredness also had important implications in the creation of the institutional settings needed for medical innovation. Long before 1792 (invasion by the revolutionary French), ruling dukes, counts, and prince-bishops had learned to live together in harmony (under the institutional forms of the Holy Roman Empire of the German Nation) and to enter into friendly competition with each other in such things as the establishment of universities. One of the latest of these was the University of Berlin, founded in 1810 through the efforts of the then Prussian minister of education, Wilhelm von Humboldt. By 1820 there were 28 universities in the German lands.

Given these favorable circumstances, the intellectual movement known as the Enlightenment took firm root in the Germanies and allied itself with Cameralism. This latter was the doctrine which held that the goal of a legitimate ruler was to work for the material betterment of his people. Cameralism also held that the real wealth of any state or principality lay in the amount, quality and variety of the material goods produced by its own inhabitants. It opposed the importation of frivolous goods and decadent ideas from overseas and was at polar odds with the laissez-faire ideology (no state interference) set forth by the Scot, Adam Smith, in his *Wealth of Nations* (1776).

Closely allied to German rulers' support for Cameralism was their conviction that in state-supported professions such as medicine, theory must ultimately ally itself with practice. In particular, this meant that men holding university degrees in medicine must begin to prove that they could actually cure people's illnesses more effectively than did the other healers on the medical marketplace. State rulers made it clear that they no longer cared to support medical doctors whose only claim to distinction was that they could spout off learnedly in Latin and Greek, and that they had the port and bearing of "gentlemen" (on the English model).

As of the 1790s, university-trained medical doctors in the German lands had many competitors. Closest to them in academic achievement were the surgeons who had attended an academy. Organized into guilds (which gave them some corporate clout) surgeons actually touched patients while sawing off arms or legs. By way of contrast, medical doctors in their old capacity of "gentlemen" never touched patients if they could possibly help it. Other fee-collecting competitors in the medical marketplace included barbers, apothecaries and drug-dealers, bath-house keepers and midwives, and itinerant empirics.

Very few German people in the eighteenth century (as opposed to the sixteenth) still resorted to magicians, white witches or the like. Even in the depths of the countryside, if rural people stayed away from university-trained medical doctors (as most of them did), it was simply because doctors' fees were too high and because their ability to effect practical cures was seen as non-existent or, at best, no better than that of any of their competitors.

At the attitudinal level, among medical students in training at the universities, the first breakthrough occurred in the 1790s with the importation of a new medical ideology coined by the obscure Scottish physician, John Brown (1735–88). Brown's followers in the German lands, called Brunians, held that the human body must be regarded as a dynamic whole. For them "life" was a dialectical process, a product of external stimuli on matter possessing "irritability." Knowledge of how this operated would lead to *the union of theory and practice* (this seems to be the first time this phrase was used). Also pregnant with meaning was the Brunians' insistence that the latest thing in French medicine, pathological anatomy, was an intellectual dead end.

The next initiative was again undertaken by princes and bureaucrats. Ever since the 1750s and 1760s, they had insisted that university medical students take a battery of examinations on practical subjects before they received their degree. It was now decreed that these exams be set and graded by outside examiners, rather than by a university's own professors (who would tend to go softly on their own students).

In the 1830s, state educational officers and princes began to insist that the practical subjects included in examinations include new bodies of knowledge such as *experimental physiology* (the study of living organisms and their body parts). In several leading universities, because of the pressure of time in a four- or five-year medical program, it was found necessary to ditch the old medical standbys – natural philosophy (i.e. Aristotle), rhetoric, pathological anatomy – in order to provide space for the conduct of controlled experiments on laboratory animals. What we have here then was the transformation of the self-image of a standard-issue medical graduate of a German university from being a "gentleman" to being the possessor of a corpus of modern scientific knowledge.

In giving pride of place to experimental physiology in the 1830s, 1840s and 1850s, it seems that the initiative was taken by authorities in Baden and in Bavaria as well as in Prussia (after 1815 by far the largest of the German states). In these polities, state officials oversaw the establishment of experimental physiology research centers at the universities of Bonn, Berlin, Leipzig, Würzburg and Heidelberg. Each center was headed by a major professor with a proven track record in research and in teaching.

The great names include Johannes Müller (1801–58) of Bonn and Berlin (author of a pioneering two-volume handbook of human physiology, published in 1833 and 1840); Karl Ludwig (1816–95) of Leipzig (author of an updated textbook on human physiology published in 1852–56); and Jacob Henle (1809–95) of Göttingen (precursor and teacher of Robert Koch). Striking off in a slightly different direction was Rudolf Virchow (1821–1902) of Berlin and Würzburg and again of Berlin, for 40 years the dominant figure in research into cells and in the medical aspects of Social Justice. Virchow never believed in germs, but instead held that poverty (malnutrition, and the like) was a direct cause of disease.

Experimental physiology, by definition, required precision in observation and in the measurement of the basic bodily functions of laboratory animals and humans. To meet its needs, appropriate equipment was devised. For example, working with skilled craftsmen in his laboratory in 1847, Karl Ludwig developed the kymograph, a machine with a rotating drum which recorded physiological happenings, such as blood pressure in arteries or veins, lung action and contractions of muscles.

Of more general applicability in the making of modern scientific medicine was the microscope. Though progress in improving upon seventeenth-century prototypes had begun in the 1830s, lens distortions persisted. Many years later, research scientists who were convinced that tiny disease-causing organisms actually existed were frustrated that they could not see them with existing laboratory equipment.

The first flowering of laboratory science

As early as 1840, Jacob Henle of Göttingen posited that infectious diseases were caused by tiny, still unseen, living organisms. Going beyond this, Henle set forth the basic rules for what (a few years later, under Koch) would become the new academic discipline of bacteriology. Drawing on what was already known about the muscarine disease of silk worms, Henle stipulated that in order to find, and to fully implicate, the specific causal agent (pathogen) it would be necessary (1) to prove that it was *always* present with the disease; (2) to isolate this causal agent in a pure culture (as would be done after 1887 with the Petri dish – a sterilized bowl invented by Koch's assistant, R. J. Petri); and (3) to reproduce the disease in a susceptible animal, using a sample from the culture. Here, in essence were the principles later know as "Koch's postulates."

Koch first demonstrated their value in 1876, when he isolated the disease causal agent of anthrax (*Bacillus anthraces*), a major killing disease among cattle that occasionally spread to humans. At the time, Koch was serving as a district medical officer in a small town in what was then eastern Germany (but now is in Poland). Like Louis Pasteur in France, Koch realized that anthrax was causing farmers huge financial loss. Using the relatively simple microscopy equipment he kept in a shed in the backyard, Koch managed to isolate and to implicate the *Bacillus anthraces* by injecting a pure culture into guinea pigs, sheep and cows, all of which promptly died. When anatomized their bodies proved to be riddled with the bacillus. Koch made his findings known to visiting professors from the University of Berlin who publicized them, thus paving the way for Koch's appointment as research scientist at the Imperial Health Institute in Berlin in 1880.

In 1881/82 Koch turned his attention to tuberculosis. At the time, TB (then variously known as consumption, phthisis, scrofula, lupus vulgaris, miliary tuberculosis) had reached epidemic proportions, especially among factory workers and slum dwellers in the rapidly growing cities of western Europe and east coast North America. During initial periods of rapid urban growth, urban TB mortality rates sometimes reached four or five per 1,000. Prevalence rates (based on the total number of cases in a given population) were, undoubtedly, very much higher.

When Koch first began his TB research in 1881, he had no idea about how complex its disease processes were. Instead he regarded his research project as a simple matter of identifying the disease causal agent. Using the famous postulates, he isolated the tubercle (taking an autopsy sample), cultivated it, injected it into a laboratory test animal, which duly died and when anatomized, was shown to be awash with tubercles. Following the requirements of modern science, Koch's experiment could be replicated anywhere by any *qualified* scientist.

"Qualified," of course, was the operative word for, in order to carry out his TB experiments, Koch almost single-handedly had to devise a complex new staining technique. This used the chemical dye, dilute alkaline methylene blue, which he smeared on his new-style pure culture media, gelatine. Then in order to differentiate the bacteria from the surrounding tissue, he counter-stained his culture with vesuvianite (a mineral). In the course of achieving his final results, which he announced to the meeting of the Berlin Physiological Society on 24 March 1882, Koch had effectively and almost single-handedly created the science of clinical bacteriology.

But having found the precise bacteria causal agent, the *Mycobacterium tuberculosis*, and cemented his reputation as Germany's (and perhaps the world's) leading medical scientist, Koch and his associates were somewhat at a loss about how best to use this knowledge. Though it was now crystal clear that TB was contagious between humans, there remained continuing uncertainty about how it spread and how it could be cured. In the event, reasonably convincing answers to these questions did not emerge until the 1950s (see Chapter 10).

Between discovery of the TB causal agent in 1882 and July 1901 (when he briefly visited medical associations in London) Koch thought deeply about these matters. He concluded that although the *Mycobacterium tuberculosis* was the *necessary* cause of TB (no bacterium, no TB), it was not the only cause. As he told British medical doctors on 21 July, diseases like it would not usually occur among people who were properly housed, properly fed, and who had reason to feel that their lives had purpose and direction. In short, by the summer of 1901, Koch had accepted an important element of Virchow's long-standing position: disease was "caused" by poverty. By this Koch meant that ill-housed, ill-nourished, ill-dressed, marginalized people were far more likely to be in positions where they would be attacked by germs and microbes than were standard middle-class people.

Beginning in the 1870s, medical students from America began to learn German so they could join the throngs of young scholars flocking to German universities. As part of their country's short-lived "Progressive Movement," they realized that the medical future lay with German-pioneered science. In the US, the first of many foundations built up on the German model was the Johns Hopkins University Medical School, in Baltimore, Maryland, founded in 1893.

English sanitary "science"

Coming out of England's long wars against France (1793 to 1815) was the gentlemanly insistence that the state should not meddle in aristocratic or middle-class persons' private affairs. This went along with the notion that out in the provinces, real authority should lie with local interest groups, headed by great landowners and gentry. The gentlemanly few also insisted that government expenditure, both at the national level, and at the local, should be kept low, and rates (taxes) minimal. Given the unreformed nature of England's *ancien regime* well into the last half of the nineteenth century, these notions closely mirrored the not particularly pleasant everyday reality experienced by ordinary people.

Another part of everyday reality, was the doubling of the size of the British population between 1800 and 1850 to number 21 million. And despite massive out-migration to America, by 1910 Britain's stay-at-home population had again doubled. Accompanying rapid population increase was rapid urbanization. By 1850, when Britain's Industrial Revolution, based on cotton, had gone into high gear, more than half the population lived in large urban settlements that statisticians defined as "cities."

Beginning as early as the 1780s, these processes occasioned widespread dislocations among agricultural and proto-industrial populations, and a great deal of unemployment and associated poverty. Calculating how best to deal with these problems on the cheap, after the end of the depression that followed the French Wars, the ruling elite had the Manchester *lawyer*, Edwin Chadwick (1800–90), create a poor-relief program. The resulting Poor Law regime (established in England in 1834) formed the basis of local government administration in medical matters until 1947 and the creation of the Welfare State.

In 1842, Chadwick and carefully selected friends released their massively influential report on the *Sanitary Condition of the Labouring Population of Great Britain*. This held that *disease caused poverty* (it will be noted that this was the precise reverse of the position that later would be held by Virchow and Koch). As far as Chadwick was concerned, the "disease causes poverty" notion meant that well-housed, well-fed, coupon-clipping middle-class people were no less likely to be struck down by "fevers" such as consumption (TB), typhus, typhoid and cholera than were ordinary members of the laboring population.

To offset this threat to respectable people, lawyer Chadwick turned to the old Greco-Roman medical notion of miasmas. As interpreted by him, this held that putrefying vegetable matter and human fecal matter released fumes (miasmas) which were the true cause of a whole range of "fever-like" diseases. The solution lay in building efficient sewerage systems which would carry these life-threatening miasmatic substances far away from built-up areas.

The Chadwickian answer to the threat posed by "fevers" thus invoked an *engineering* solution to the nation's disease problems, rather than a solution which required the expertise of medical doctors. Government endorsement of Chadwick's idea of "sanitary science" was one of the reasons why after 1854, the avant-garde research of John Snow into cholera and its transmission through water contaminated with cholera-bearing human fecal matter received so little official recognition.

Long after the era of Chadwick (forced out of public life in 1854), the British medical profession remained a two-tiered affair. At the top were the gentlemanly physicians who had been educated at Oxford or Cambridge, very much in the old style. Gentlemanly physicians built up their practice among a well-heeled clientele by acquiring a reputation for their pleasing bed-side manners, and in behaving and dressing as gentlemen, complete with frock coats, gold-topped canes and carriages. In this patient-centered system (which had close parallels with what pertained among high-class medical professionals in China before 1840 and in India before 1757), each fee-paying patron's disease condition was considered to be "unique."

Failed attempts to establish a national public health system

Yet by the 1860s, attempts were being made to establish rational guidelines for a yet-to-be-born public health department which was envisaged as having legally enforceable authority throughout the kingdom. A key figure in the endeavor was Dr John Simon (1816–1904), Medical Officer to the Privy Council from 1858 to 1871, then chief Medical Officer of the Local Government Board until 1875 (when he finally threw in the towel).

Simon's first great achievement was to learn the skills needed to massage the egos of the gentleman capitalists who controlled England. Realizing that they wanted everything done on the cheap and that the miasmic theory of disease causation (local smells caused disease) beautifully suited this purpose, he generally worded his statements in a way which could be interpreted as meaning that he endorsed miasmatic causation. Yet, in his actions, Simon proceeded in a way that showed he fully accepted the germ theory of disease causation which had been set forth by John Snow in 1849 and 1854 (in his publications on cholera) and more recently by William Budd (of Bristol) in his publications on typhoid.

Most of John Simon's work in public health was done on the national level. After he retired in 1875, there was little progress at that level for many years (indeed, the founding of a ministry of health was delayed until 1911 – a time lag of 36 years). However, Simon was also instrumental in achieving effective influence for the *local level* agencies (the Poor Law Union level, Medical Officers of Health) which had been created in incoherent form in 1848. Through his work in and after 1866, Simon, in company with Town Hall administrators, was able to ensure that the inhabitants of urban Victorian England would not again be worked over by waves of epidemic disease.

Thus, in the wake of England's last major epidemic of cholera imported from overseas in 1866, Simon had surveys made of the biological quality of the water supplied to customers of London's various private water companies. Some companies were shown to be consistently infecting their customers with cholera (then still a hypothesized germ, which Koch would definitively identify under his microscope in Calcutta in 1884). Simon (and gentlemen of influence upstairs) forced these water companies to clean up their act.

Working on the broader scene, Simon saw to it that special Medical Officers of Health were installed at the Port of London and at England's other ports of entry. These officials rigorously inspected incoming passengers and crew, checking for cholera and other infectious diseases. People who did not show disease symptoms, but had come from places where cholera was known to exist, were kept under medical supervision (this meant they could go home, but had to report in regularly to a health office until they could be certified as safe, non-carriers).

Simon also oversaw the establishment of the legal requirement that local health authorities be *notified* of any outbreak of infectious disease. Going along with medical *surveillance* and notification was the establishment of *isolation* units for certified infectious disease bearers. In London, hulks (demasted ships) stationed in the Thames served this purpose. Using these techniques, infected individuals were prevented from setting off an epidemic which might kill hundreds of victims.

Nibbling away at the consciences of England's top people, John Simon, together with Joseph Chamberlain the mayor of Birmingham, Charles Dickens (through his novels), and other influential reformers saw to it that, from the 1870s onwards, the Town Fathers of festering new industrial cities came to *vie with each other* in the provision of decent sewerage systems, water supply systems and other sanitary improvements. As Simon Szreter has so ably shown, in England it was at the *local municipal level* that the basic quality-of-life improvements were made which, from the 1870s onwards, finally permitted the average English or Welsh person's expectation of life at birth to increase from age 40 (where it was in 1841 and had been for 20 years) to 51.5 by 1911. Even in London (since Tudor times, a sink-hole of death for immigrants from the rest of England) average life expectancy at birth rose from 35 in 1841 to almost 40 in 1911.

These improvements in municipal sanitation cost vast sums of money, much of which was borrowed, on favorable terms, from the central government. Again quoting Szreter's figures, local government spending on sanitary improvements rose from around £5 million a year in the period 1856–71, to around £12–14 million a year in the period 1874–94, to around £30 million a year in the period 1901–10. Making this possible, loans or subventions from the central Treasury to municipal governments increased from 6.7 percent of total UK revenue in 1890, to 11.6 percent of total revenue in 1913.

In short, if "the proof of the pudding is in the eating" the United Kingdom was able to keep abreast (or indeed, slightly in advance of) recently unified Germany in lengthening the life expectancies of its inhabitants and in cutting down mortality rates, especially from infectious diseases. In Germany, the mortality rate in 1901–10 was 18.7 per 1,000. In England and Wales it was marginally less: 15.4 per 1,000.

Empire and medicine: India

By odd coincidence, the sum that Szreter found the British national government made available each year to urban authorities for sanitary improvements in the period 1874–94 (£12–£14 million p.a.) was very similar to the sum (£15–£16 million p.a.) paid over annually in the same period by the people of India to the London government and to UK investors in Indian development projects. The same odd coincidence was apparent between 1901–10, when the £30 million annually made available by Central Government to English cities for sanitary improvements was, again, just a bit *less* than the amount annually taken from the people of India to be sent to England in the form of "home charges," returns on investment, payment on outstanding "debt," tribute from Native Princes and the like.

Perhaps too much should not be read into these particular figures and coincidences. Accordingly, let us approach the Indian health and financial situation from another direction, using little-used primary source material in the India Office (in London).

Here, for example, we find that in 1898 two Indian members of the All-India budget review committee meeting in Simla (the capital) reminded the Viceroy to his face that India was currently being drained of its supplies of hard cash to pay for (1) British-engineered frontier wars; (2) the maintenance of one of the world's largest standing armies (stationed in India, consisting largely of Indians); and (3) payment of "debts" outstanding in England (i.e. interest due to gentleman venture capitalists on investment in development).

The Indian members went on to state that if the money now being drained out of India were, instead, spent on building up its infrastructure, it would soon be able to create modern public health and disease-control facilities. With facilities of this sort (which the Raj had yet to sanction – indeed, it never did) India would be able to bring under control the epidemics of cholera, malaria and bubonic plague currently washing over the country, virtually unopposed. Given that this was the situation in 1898 (worse was to come in 1900) it is appropriate to identify some of the steps which had led up to this dire state of affairs.

Eighty years earlier, one of the first acts of the conquering British had been to confiscate the landed endowments that had long supported Unani Tibb training academies. In addition to cutting off the life-blood of Unani Tibb and Ayurvéda recruitment programs, early nineteenth-century British administrators had also rearranged local village hierarchies.

In the past (under the Mughals), a system of voluntary contributions had paid the wages of the sweepers who had always kept villages clean. But under the dictate of British revenue officers, these customary assessments were now raked in and (in a manner of speaking) sent off to the UK Treasury. As a result, under the Raj, Indian villages were left unswept.

Professing to be unaware that this situation was a creation of Raj revenue collection policies, after 1868 most British health officials claimed that Indian villages had been awash with human and animal fecal matter from "time immemorial." By falling back on this Orientalist argument, upper echelon British health officers thought to exonerate themselves of any responsibility for sanitary conditions in village India. Yet in fact, the *non-provision* of sanitation and potable water in rural India was one of the defining characteristics of British policy. This brings us to a second characteristic: consistent British denial after 1868 of the findings of modern medical science.

Until the late 1860s, British medical doctors who were in India to tend to the health needs of British officials and soldiers were under no compulsion to uphold ideas about disease causation that were any different in kind from those generally held by enlightened members of the medical profession in mainland Europe and the British Isles. This held true for *cholera* as well as for many other diseases.

Until mid-1868, the general consensus of medical men and civil officers in India (as reported by the unbiased Inspector-General of Hospitals, John Murray) was that cholera was much as John Snow had described it back in 1849 and 1854. It was caused by some sort of germ, which infected the human gut where it proliferated and then was expelled in human fecal matter. If this fecal matter entered a drinking water supply it was likely to cause an epidemic outbreak of cholera – with a case-mortality of upwards of 50 percent.

Building on this insight, at an international conference of cholera experts held in Constantinople in 1866 at which English and Scottish doctors from India were present, it was decided that movement of cholera could best be blocked by preventing the movement of suspect cholera carriers. This could be done through the use of *quarantine* procedures against ships at sea, and the use of *cordon sanitaire* against the movement of suspect people on land. The conference also strongly recommended that all cholera sick be isolated in special hospitals, given that the disease was likely to infect any attendant who happened to come into contact with infected fecal matter. This was in 1866.

However, in the last months of 1868, on the eve of the opening of the Suez Canal, the freedom of British medical doctors in India to keep purely medical considerations uppermost in mind came to an abrupt end. At that time, influential members of the governing elite in London (including some gentleman venture capitalists) decided that they could not permit the new-style British steamships which had been purpose-built for the run back and forth between Bombay and London to be delayed by quarantine procedures at the entrance to the Suez Canal. Given that the newly created route cut the time and distance necessary to sail between Bombay and London in half (compared to the old route around the Cape), and that time was money – measurable in terms of coaling costs, crew hire costs and the like – ten or more days spent in quarantine at Suez would massively cut down profits accruing to shipping companies and investors.

At the Suez Canal, quarantine procedures would be enforced by an international quarantine commission which Britain was not always able to control – it never had hegemonic power over all other nations in the world. In part for this reason (and in part because the UK considered itself the world's most civilized state), Britain was highly sensitive to foreign criticism. Thus, in 1868 the governing elite in London thought it essential to come up with a new medical (or pseudo-scientific) interpretation of the principal disease against which quarantine procedures would be applied: cholera.

The Edinburgh medical man they would appoint at the end of the year to head their *non-interventionist* campaign was, at first sight, a curious choice, given that until recently he seemed to be one of the leading proponents of *interventionist* measures. In 1867, a few months after the Constantinople conference, James McNabb Cuningham (1829–1905) was temporarily serving as the chief sanitary official in India. When cholera struck and raged across northern India, Cuningham had dutifully applied all the techniques suggested by the Constantinople conference. Using *cordon sanitaire*, isolation hospitals and quarantines he had successfully prevented epidemic cholera from entering the large cities and causing a disease holocaust. Cuningham then sent a full report of what he had done to London.

However, just at this time in London, governing elites were in the final stages of creating a new interpretation of cholera in India which would rule out the need for quarantine at Suez or the use of *cordon sanitaire*, notification, isolation or surveillance. To this end, they did something straight out of Machiavelli's *The Prince* (manual of statecraft). They appointed James McNabb Cuningham as full, permanent, chief sanitary officer in India with authority to dismiss any health official who dared to question their new cholera interpretation.

Cuningham (with his upgraded pay and pension schedule in hand) immediately set to work. His new interpretation held that "experience . . . has again and again testified to the truth of the conclusion that cholera is *not* carried by persons from one locality to another." From this it of course followed that the quarantining of ships to prevent the movement of infected persons from say Bombay to Suez and on to London, was entirely unnecessary.

In 1868/69 the then Secretary of State for India and the rest of Britain's governing elite were well aware that foreign nations might not accept the truth of assertions of the sort made by chief sanitary commissioner James Cuningham unless they were backed up with the findings of what could be claimed to be "science." Accordingly, they appointed two other individuals to assist Cuningham in his work. One was the young research scientist, Douglas Cunningham (who we will turn to in a moment); the other was James Bryden (1833–80). It was Bryden who, in 1868, cobbled together the central tenets of the new anti-quarantine, anti-interventionist doctrine.

According to Bryden, cholera was a type of miasma which was carried by the wind; from this it of course followed that its movement could not be blocked by quarantines and *cordon sanitaire*. Then, abruptly shifting from a fifth-century BCE "Airs, Waters, Places" interpretation of disease to an approach pioneered in Britain in the seventeenth century CE, Bryden claimed that the movement of cholera always followed regular patterns. If properly recorded over time, these patterns could be reduced to statistical observations.

Thereafter, Government used Bryden's statistical approach to the understanding of cholera as one of its principal tools to smother the germ theory of disease. Working through the agency of the Chief Sanitary Commissioner with the Government of India, James McNabb Cuningham, the Army Sanitary Commission in London and Florence Nightingale (of Crimean War fame), Government claimed that the *non-communicability* of cholera was an established *fact* and that any attempt to prove otherwise was mere theorizing. To go out to a cholera-stricken village and to examine the village water supply and to discover it contained human fecal matter and then to decide that the two situations were connected, was to engage in the sin of "theorizing." Confronted with this Government dictum about "facts" and "theory," most young medical men in India conformed, lest they lose their jobs and be sent home to an England where there was a glut of medical school graduates awaiting jobs.

Yet a few, now forgotten, long-experienced medical officers did not conform: one of these was M. C. Furnell, between 1879 and 1884, sanitary commissioner for the vast province of Madras in southern India. Furnell was actively engaged in what Government called "theorizing" in 1881 when he went to the nearby French enclave at Pondicherry and found that the French had overseen the provision of protected water supplies in each village. Because Pondicherry's well-constructed wells could not be contaminated by human fecal matter, there was no cholera in these villages even though there was plenty of cholera in English-controlled territories nearby.

In a second bout of "theorizing," early in 1884, Furnell met personally with Robert Koch when the German scientist passed nearby on his way to Calcutta and its famous cholera-tanks at which he conclusively proved that the cholera vibrio contained in human fecal matter was the one and only causal agent of cholera.

Later in 1884 (in such things, there was considerable time-lag) Furnell's "theorizing" activities in 1881 were brought to the attention of the House of Commons in London. He was accused of writing an annual report which, by endorsing the germ theory, had provided the International Quarantine authorities at Alexandria and Constantinople with information they had immediately used to put British shipping coming from Bombay into quarantine. In the event, this 1881 quarantine measure was not still in force in 1883. In that year, ships coming from cholera-pestered Bombay introduced the disease in epidemic form into Egypt. Sweeping southward from the Canal all the way to Aswan (and northwards to Alexandria) it caused upwards of 60,000 deaths, a mortality rate of 8.95 per 1,000.

While Egyptian events were in the last stages of working themselves out (through the sorting out of investigation committee reports and the like), Furnell was in Britain where he delivered a scathing speech in which he attacked the "unintelligible" cholera policies for India which Government insisted were "the one true faith." A few months later he died under peculiar circumstances.

This brings us back to the third of the trio of experts Government employed in 1868 in order to establish "the one true faith": this was the young research scientist, Douglas Cunningham (1843–1914). Brought to India to demonstrate, through the use of his microscope, that no mainstream European or US interpretation of cholera was relevant to India, Douglas Cunningham was still at his post in 1897, teaching at the Calcutta Medical School and publishing anti-quarantine, anti-interventionist tracts. In his very last publication (1897) he re-asserted for the umpteenth time that Koch's vibrio was not the cause of cholera, that human fecal matter did not carry a cholera causal agent, and that water carrying fecal matter did not cause cholera.

Ten years earlier, at the International Congress of Hygiene and Demography held in Vienna (1887), delegates severely castigated Great Britain for her neglect of basic sanitary matters in India. One of the papers read at the Congress was by Florence Nightingale (1820–1910). A short time later, Nightingale followed this up with a letter to the Secretary of State for India in which she asserted that "the unsanitary condition of Indian villages is undermining the health of the rural population."

Government was somewhat taken aback by an attack coming from this direction. Ever since 1868, Nightingale had been a firm supporter of the notion that cholera was not at all a contagious disease and that quarantine procedures to control its movement were evil. Though she maintained the fiction that she was an invalid who could not leave her rooms in South Street, London (just off Park Lane), over the years Nightingale had managed to entice leading officials from the War Office, the India Office, and the Government of India, into her residence, where she hectored them about the incompetence of modern doctors who insisted on doing laboratory research. As far as she was concerned all the "facts" about cholera were already known. As she pointed out in an article in *The Lancet* in 1870, there was no need to waste public money doing further research on the disease.

Given that Nightingale was a national icon who was tremendously well connected, in 1887/88, 17 years after her *Lancet* blast, Government felt it had to be seen to be paying heed to her claim that the health of India's rural population was being undermined by unsanitary conditions of the sort which it was within the power of any proper government to correct. Accordingly, the Secretary of State for India sent her letter on to the Governor General who in turn sent it to all the principal officials in charge of public health in India, asking for their comments.

These 20 or so responses (all available in the Records of the India Office in London) are of some interest. For its part the Government of India replied that although its achievements in sanitary affairs had, thus far, been "small," its first priority, when it came to spending funds, was to "open up the internal resources of the country by means of improved communications." This meant that money would be made available for roads, telegraphs and posts, but not for matters of *secondary* importance, such as sanitation in rural India. In short the needs of "development" came first.

For his part, the Surgeon Major of Bombay, J. Pinkerton, stated that the high death rate in Indian villages was not due to the non-existence of sanitation, but rather to the "racial composition of the population." Summing up all the comments found in the returns, H. H. Fowler (of Simla) felt able to assert that "to say, as is said in [Nightingale's] memorandum that present insanitary condition of the villages are undermining the health of rural populations seems to be using the language of exaggeration." Nightingale's feeble reply (she was then in her mid-seventies) suggests that she knew she had been put in her place.

Then in September 1889, the son and heir of T. G. Hewlett succeeded in having Government print a pamphlet written by his late father. Beginning in 1867, T. G. Hewlett had been an active agent in managing the health affairs of the city of Bombay. He had first served as the city health officer, then become sanitary commissioner for the province of Bombay, a post he held until his retirement in 1888.

Writing about rural health and sanitation in the province which served as Britain's gateway into India, Hewlett's conclusions speak for themselves:

> it is a matter of the utmost certainty [that if village India were provided with sanitation and water] cholera would at once lose its intensity and eventually become eradicated . . . a healthier rural population would grow up . . . the labour market would be more amply supplied . . . and the revenue of the country would be augmented, while England would cease to be, as now, stigmatized by foreign nations as being entirely indifferent to the just demands of the civilized world to the real welfare of the 200 million of natives of India committed to its charge among whom such a terrible mortality is now permitted year after year to take place without any measures being taken by Government to prevent it.
>
> (Hewlett 1888)

That was the state of affairs in 1888. After that the situation worsened. In the single year, 1900, nearly a million Indians died of cholera in the famine-relief work camps set up by a government which had yet to learn anything about disease control.

Writing in 1921, soon after the Government of India sought to cut costs by handing over responsibility for public health to financially starved, locally elected bodies in the provinces, the Director of Public Health in Madras, A. J. H. Russell, stated that: "Little has been done in the past as regards investigation of the epidemiology of infectious disease. . . . The methods adapted at present are in most instances *primitive and unscientific* and as a consequence are entirely inadequate to meet the requirements of the situation."

Two and a half decades later, on the eve of Independence in 1947, a study commission reported that life expectancy in England had *risen* to well over 50. However, in India it had steadily *fallen* from 24.59 years in 1891, to 23.63 in 1901, to 22.59 in 1911 and to only 20.1 in 1921. By 1947, it had fallen even further. These then were the fruits of "development," British-style.

Further reading

On Germany: Thomas H. Broman, *The Transformation of German Academic Medicine, 1750–1820* (Cambridge University Press, 1995); Claudia Huerkamp, "The Making of the Modern Medical Profession, 1800–1914: Prussian doctors in the nineteenth century," in Geoffrey Cocks and Konrad H. Jarausch (eds) *German Professions, 1800–1950* (Oxford University Press, 1990), 66–84; Arleen Tuchman, *Science, Medicine, and the State in Germany: the case of Baden, 1815–1871* (Oxford University Press, 1993); Brian Bracegirdle, "The Microscopical Tradition," in Roy Porter and William Bynum (eds) *Companion Encyclopedia of the History of Medicine* (Routledge, 1993), 102–19. A detailed overview of English medicine: Roy Porter, *The Greatest Benefit to Mankind* (HarperCollins, 1997), 245–492. An important revisionist account: Steve Sturdy and Roger Cooter, "Science, Scientific Management, and the Transformation of Medicine in Britain *c.* 1870–1950," *History of Science* xxxvi (1998), 421–66. For a conceptual breakthrough on the role of public health: Simon Szreter, "The Importance of Social Intervention in Britain's Mortality Decline *c.* 1850–1914: a re-interpretation of the role of public health," *The Society for the Social History of Medicine*, vol. 1 nos. 1, 2, 3 (1988), 1–37. On the transformation of British medicine in India: Sheldon Watts, "From Rapid Change to Stasis: official responses to cholera in British-ruled India and Egypt: 1800 to *c.* 1921," *Journal of World History* vol. 12, no 2 (2001), 321–74; Sheldon Watts, "British Development Policies and Malaria in India 1897–*c.* 1929," *Past & Present* no. 165, November 1999, 141–81. Cambridge University History website: www.historyand policy.org/.

Chapter 10

Health and medicine in the world, 1940 to the present

Introductory thoughts

In 1981, medical scientists discovered a highly contagious, heretofore unknown disease that was striking down large numbers of sexually active young adult men and women: it was called AIDS (acquired immune deficiency syndrome). Later it was decided that this new-found presence was spread by a virus termed HIV (human immunodeficiency virus). No less disturbing was the finding that certain pathogens – such as those of tuberculosis and malaria – were in the process of mutating to become immune to the drugs that scientists had earlier devised to kill them off.

Yet on the credit side of the ledger, the most important happening from the mid-1940s onwards was the new-found *ability* of modern Western medicine to cure a wide range of acute infectious diseases through the application of an increasingly wide range of therapies. There has also been a massive expansion in the Western knowledge base about the workings of the human body – the heretofore unknown existence of its *immune system* for example. There is also new knowledge about disease causal agents. We are now aware, for instance, that *viruses* are altogether different from bacteria: unlike them they are totally host-dependent.

In the developed countries in the North (where, at the time of writing, 15 percent of the world's population live – the US share being only 4.5 percent), going along with this very real progress in the years after the Second World War was a reconceptualization of what formal-sector medical services were all about. Gone were the days when the family doctor came to a sick person's house to offer advice on how to cope, knowing that he had no way to cure the patient. Nowadays, in the world's North, the formal medical sector is based on high-tech hospitals, with their laboratories, technicians, managerial staff and cost accountants. In these new-style institutions, the patient (unless she or he is a celebrity) tends to be reduced to the status of a depersonalized sufferer from disease "x" and is treated as a "case" rather than as an "individual."

Among ethnic majority peoples living in the world's North, (Europeans, Euro-Americans, Japanese) the last half of the twentieth century saw the "epidemiologic transition." This refers to the massive *decline* in the percentage of a given population that died of infectious diseases in early childhood or before the age of 50, and the great increase in the number of people who, in middle and old age, suffered from chronic disease conditions – heart trouble, cardiovascular problems, diabetes, cancers of various sorts. Accompanying increased longevity – women commonly living into their mid-eighties and men into their early eighties – there was a great increase in the numbers of sufferers from the degenerative diseases of old age (such as Alzheimer's).

In World Historical terms, the development of increasingly high proportions of total population in the West who were over the age of 65 was unprecedented. So, too, was the steady and apparently permanent *decline* in the overall percentage of young adults who were prepared to undergo the rigors of parenthood. Instead, it was increasingly common to regard sexual activity as a recreation rather than as a means of perpetuating the species. As a result, in Germany and some other mainland European countries, at the time of writing, overall population is shrinking. To offset the decline in the proportion of persons of working-age who fund the pension schemes drawn on by the aged, some experts recommend bringing in young, highly trained professional people from the world's South. Here then, even in human terms the South is seen as a resource base for the North.

At the beginning of the twenty-first century, the situation in the Nonwest (where 85 percent of the world's population live) was less clear cut. It was known, however, that in a middle range less developed country, like Egypt, more than 48 million people (out of its total population of 70 million) did not make much use of the formal medical system. Instead, they made do as best they could with non-standard medical assistance and with Western drugs (or their locally produced equivalent) purchased over a druggist's counter. It is instructive to sort out why this was so.

In theory, in the wake of throwing out the British (the Free Officers' Revolution of 1952), Egyptians were provided with free, government-sponsored urban and rural health facilities located within a few kilometers of every citizen's home. Yet in practice, after the mid-1980s, these facilities were subjected to severe budgetary constraints. Among other things, staff salaries were pegged at levels which bore no relation to rising costs of living for middle-class professional doctors with families to support. According to official statistics, only 1.7 percent of Egypt's GNP is spent on health: this compares to the 15 percent of GNP spent on health in the US. This vast difference in levels of spending is reflected at hospital bed-sides. In Egypt reliable 24-hours a day nursing care for patients simply does not exist, whereas in middle America, family members know that the nursing needs of their loved one will be attended to, at the ring of the bed-side bell, day or night.

Medical-cultural historians are aware of the creative uses to which statistics can be put. They are also aware that the World Bank (based in Washington DC) and the International Monetary Fund (an agency of the United Nations) were founded with the understanding that they should further "development" (defined in Chapter 7), and that since 1980 they have played a dominant role in matters pertaining to the health of the Non-western world. Cultural historians are also aware that the World Bank and IMF are under the direction of economists who uphold a certain ideology. This holds that the provision of health facilities should be considered to be a commodity like any other and that users should pay a "fair market price" for services. World Bank and IMF ideology also holds that services provided by private enterprise are, by definition, superior to those provided by the state. None of these claims can be scientifically verified.

As it happened, in the 1960s and 1970s, heads of government in most of the nation states in newly de-colonized Africa and in Latin America (liberated from Spain in the 1810s and 1820s) allowed themselves to be persuaded to have their governments borrow vast sums of money from American and European banks to fund the "development" projects which (if completed) would demonstrate the full modernity of their countries. Interest payments on these loans were to be in US dollars or equivalent "hard currency."

These requirements put debtor nations in a dangerously exposed position which 500 years of colonialism, globalization, and fiscal exploitation at the hands of the Dutch, the French and the English should have warned them against. However, Non-western nations tended to be ruled by technocrats and military men who were products of colonial-inspired educational systems which ignored these elementary lessons from the past.

The coming of worldwide recession in the 1980s hit debtor nations very hard, particularly because most of them had directed their economies to the production of primary products (such as cocoa, coffee and cotton) for export to the world's North, rather than to the foodstuffs needed by their own populations to prevent them from becoming seriously malnourished. It is now known that malnutrition has an almost immediate negative impact on people's immune systems. The malnourished readily fall prey to cholera, pneumonia, TB and other acute infectious diseases that the immune system of a standard-issue well-fed person can usually shrug off.

In the 1980s, in an effort to preserve their credit ratings, debtor nations (including Egypt) turned to the World Bank and the IMF asking to be bailed out so they could make timely repayment of interest due. In exchange for bail-outs, they accepted IMF and World Bank Structural Adjustment Programs (SAPs). Following these guidelines, they gave priority to maintaining existing development projects, to paying interest on their debt and to cutting back on social services such as health and education.

By 1985, Latin American countries caught up in the clutches of the IMF and the World Bank were making hard currency transfers to external creditors in the amount of US$35 billion *more* than they were receiving in further loans to maintain existing development projects and social services.

A few years later, following the collapse of the old USSR (in 1989) and the end of the threat to the West of global Communism, the flow of capital for debt repayment *to* the rich from the world's poorest nations was $178 billion a year: less than $61 billion went in the other direction.

Meddlings by rich nations in health matters in the world's South have had mixed results. Already by the 1920s, the smallpox vaccination campaigns which Raj authorities in India insisted should replace old-style indigenous inoculation as a preventive measure had led to a substantial increase in the number of children who stayed alive long enough to have children of their own. In the event, India's population increase was matched by rapidly falling life expectancies at birth (see Chapter 9).

With the coming of Independence (India 1947, Ghana 1957, Nigeria 1960 and so on) the political leaders of new nation states were able to pick and choose which aspects of their former colonial masters' culture they would keep (and try to enlarge upon) and which aspects they would reject. Among the cultural practices most of them decided to reject were birth control, family limitation and homosexuality. These were seen as elements in white men's conspiracy to achieve demographic hegemony over the world. Today, most ordinary people in the Non-west regard marriage as the normative condition to which everyone should aspire, and that the main purpose of marriage is the procreation of children.

In the Non-west after 1977 (and the worldwide abolition of smallpox as a free-ranging disease), contributing further to rapid population growth were World Health Organization programs directed toward improving the well-being of mothers and infants. Putting to use new knowledge about the role of specific vaccines, huge numbers of Non-western children were vaccinated against the old childhood killers – measles, tetanus, diphtheria, whooping cough, poliomyelitis and tuberculosis. In addition, WHO agents supported efforts to instruct ordinary health providers in the use of the simple equipment needed for oral rehydration – thus preventing infant diarrhea from taking its usual toll of young lives.

As a result of these interventions huge numbers of infants, who in the old days would have died early, survived to young adulthood, married, and had children of their own. In 1950 (before interventions began) there were 2.5 billion people in the world, an increase of 64 percent over the number found in 1901 (1.6 billion). Fifty years later, in 2001, the 2.5 billion had increased by 240 percent to number some 6.1 billion souls. Currently, in most Non-western countries nearly half the population are *below* the age of 15, too young to hold down responsible jobs; less than 4 percent are over the age of 65.

As of 2002, 1.2 billion people, a fifth of the world's population, were living in "extreme poverty," defined as having access to less than two US dollars a day. Nearly 2,400,000,000 lacked access to sanitation, without which the maintenance of good health is nearly impossible.

In the year 2001, the citizens of the US (with an average per capita income of $26,980) were spending 15 percent of their GNP on health care. However, according to figures R. Guerrant made available from 1997, the US (with its population of 260 million) was spending only one-tenth of one percent (0.001%) of its GNP on development assistance to less fortunate countries ($7.3 billion). This amount was far behind the actual sum spent by Japan ($14 billion, Japan's population was 122 million), or France ($8.4 billion, population 54 million), or Germany ($7.5 billion, population 77 million).

On the other hand, as of 1997, more than 60 percent of the oil and such like of the world's non-renewable resources were being consumed by the 15 percent of the global population who lived in the developed countries (the North). Medical historians also note that in the year 2000, when the United Kingdom (the creator of the Modern World System and at one time the world's largest colonial power) was giving out US$ 3.2 billion in development "aid" (variously defined – some of it was in the form of army personnel carriers), the pre-tax profits of the UK-based pharmaceutical company GlaxoSmithKlein amounted to $8,000,000,000 (two and a half times the sum given in "aid").

Yet the health care divide between rich and poor is not delineated by the boundaries of nation states. Even within the richest of the countries in the world – the free-enterprise US – there are pockets of acute misery. According to figures released in September 2002, the number of Americans living in "poverty" has now risen to 32,700,000. Many of those in poverty are African Americans living in non-fashionable parts of New York and other large cities. For them, a common cause of death has come to be drug-resistant TB (the poverty disease par excellence).

Moreover, at the beginning of the twenty-first century, 40 percent of the US population were not protected by any form of health insurance. This meant that the country's free-enterprise hospitals and clinics were closed to them unless they could prove they had absolutely no assets and were given admittance in their capacity as "deserving poor."

The rich/poor division is also found in the Non-west. In all the poor nations of the world there exists a small elite who are able to acquire the best of everything leading to good health, either locally (from under the counter or from reserves in the Presidential Palace) or at the other end of an airline flight to a metropolis in the West.

The disputed role of preventive medicine

In 1976, Thomas McKeown (a Canadian physician living in England) published a highly contentious book in which he claimed that the lengthening life expectancies which earlier historical demographers had found existed in Europe and North America after 1880 owed nothing at all to the interventions of medical doctors. McKeown's savage attack on the competence of physicians and surgeons to cure an actual disease (such as the influenza which killed off 21 million people worldwide in 1918–19) led to a new appraisal and a reaffirmation of the role of "sanitary improvements" in the making of a healthier Europe and Euro-America after 1880.

As we saw in Chapter 9, by "sanitation" was meant municipal and regional government provision of safe drinking water and of compulsory household connection to sewerage systems. As a result, people no longer needed to live near streets and alleys awash with human fecal matter. More broadly defined, "sanitation" also meant slum clearance and controls on food processing techniques and the like.

In 1978, moving on from consensual agreement on the vital role played by "sanitation" in promoting "good health" – and in recognition of the recent birth of new nations in Asia and Africa following "decolonization" – health ministers from all over the world met at Alma Ata in the then Soviet Union. There they agreed that it was essential (from the point of view of our common humanity) that every person in the world be given access to primary health care facilities. PHC facilities – particularly in the case of the Non-west – were seen as a first line of defense against the outbreak of illnesses, rather than as curative centers for major diseases.

It was envisioned that this preventive mission would be carried out through early detection and surveillance, through the provision of vaccines (to provide immunity to old killer diseases), and through teaching mothers about oral rehydration to suppress childhood diarrhea. In 1979, the general meeting of the World Health Organization approved the Alma Ata Declaration and launched its program of "Health for All by the year 2000."

These were the years of optimism when everything seemed possible. Marking the successful conclusion of the WHO campaign begun 20 years earlier with funding from the USSR, later topped up with $300 million from America, in 1977 the WHO was able to announce the abolition of smallpox (as found in nature). As we saw in Chapter 7, in the years after 1518, smallpox had been one of the (if not *the* principal) killing disease which had wiped out most of the indigenous population of the Americas. Since then it had become a major threat to children and adults worldwide. The eradication of smallpox in 1977 (except for the laboratory samples US government anti-terrorists experts insisted, as late as 2003, be kept on hand in storage vaults in Atlanta, Georgia) is the *one* clear example of a disease which has been exterminated by human agency.

But as of the year 2003, humanity (particularly in the Non-west) continued to suffer the ill-effects of another WHO campaign – the failed attempt to eradicate malaria in Asia, Latin America and three countries in Africa (in the rest of Africa, the predominant forms of malaria were regarded as intractable, so no attempt at their eradication was made). The sorry tale began in the late 1950s when WHO officials let themselves believe that by killing off all malaria-hosting mosquitoes by the liberal use of DDT (dichloro-diphenyl-trichloroethane) on agricultural lands and villages, they could break the chain of insect hosts the *plasmodia* causal agent needed in order to perpetuate itself. It was also hoped that by the ingestion of chloroquine and other quinine-derived pills (taken daily or weekly) humans who were hosting one or more of the various forms of *plasmodia* in their blood would be cleared of the disease.

Unfortunately, WHO planners did not take into account local bureaucratic failure to repeatedly spray mosquito-prone areas season after season and so to kill off *all* potential DDT-proof mutants before they did mutate. They also did not take into account long distance migration by people carrying malaria in their blood, or Western funders' (the US Congress) waning interest (malaria had all but disappeared from North America and Northern Europe by 1930). WHO also failed to take heed of Raj medical men's warnings dating from as early as 1911 that *plasmodia* causal agents in India might mutate and become resistant to quinine and its derivatives.

The results of program failure were abundantly clear by 1977. Now sweeping anew over much of the Non-west were malarial forms which were immune to standard prophylactic techniques and to old-style cures. Adding to the difficulty was the Western discovery that DDT killed off all sorts of other living things in addition to malarial mosquitoes. Accordingly, a massive campaign against all further use of DDT for *any* purpose anywhere in the world was launched by a well-meaning American woman, Rachel Carlson. Her pace setting book, *Silent Spring*, set the tone for the emerging Green Movement which protested against the assaults of mainstream science on "nature," regarded as unchanging and benign.

In retrospect it can been seen that the vision conjured up by the WHO in 1979 of "Health for All by the Year 2000" through the provision of Primary Health Care (PHC) centers in every corner of the globe ran against the spirit of the age. In the first place, in the Non-west PHC staffing requirements did not favor fast-track, career-oriented, young persons being trained in medical schools – on the late nineteenth-century German model – to think of themselves as laboratory scientists, or at the very least as practitioners who would have easy access to the diagnostic certainties of a laboratory. Instead of expensively educated personnel like this, PHC facilities required only slightly updated versions of the Barefooted Doctors who were being touted by Communist China as marvelously successful in improving the health of its half billion peasant farmers.

And in addition to its negative appeal to young medical students worldwide, the PHC movement (designed for the poor) ran afoul of the managerial technocrat class who saw their own (high-pay) career futures as being tied up with the creation of huge urban hospital complexes modeled on famous institutions such as the Mayo Clinic in Rochester, Minnesota. By the early 1960s (in exchange for big money) the Mayo Clinic was offering treatment for the new range of chronic diseases of old age – cancer, heart ailments, cardiovascular problems. Much of the big money required for these enterprises was channeled through increasingly powerful health and life insurance companies with head offices in Hartford, Connecticut and other finance centers.

Also incompatible with Primary Health Care facilities in the Non-west (where hardly anyone had much in the way of ready cash) were the requirements of another breed of for-profit organizations, the great pharmaceutical companies, based in Germany, Switzerland, Britain and the US. These firms claimed they needed huge sums to engage in cutting-edge laboratory research into cures of proven effectiveness which they could patent (against competitors) and then sell on the world market for great sums.

By the year 2002, some of these firms were creating "cures" for natural conditions such as baldness and then proclaiming on TV that these natural conditions were actually illnesses. By creating a "cure" for what until then had never been considered a disease, it was intended that huge profits could be made. Meanwhile, in the world as a whole, 2,400,000,000 people did not have access to "sanitation" and certainly could not afford to buy any laboratory-tested drug at a "fair market" price.

Medicine's positive achievements after 1940 and their antecedents

Among Euro-American and allied western European voters and taxpayers, the medical profession was *not* accepted as an essential part of modern society until it was perceived to have achieved significant curative breakthroughs; this perceptual change occurred in the 1940s and 1950s. Of the perceived curative breakthroughs, the most important was doubtless the creation of the first effective antibiotic – penicillin – in 1941, and its mass production and highly successful application on the war wounds of Anglo-American and Free French troops in Algeria and Morocco early in 1943.

Yet the creation of antibiotics did not come out of a short-term, politically motivated, funding blitz. Instead, it was the result of patient laboratory research that had been going on for decades. Half a century earlier, medical scientists had realized that certain aspects of the Hobbesian world of bacteria (the timeless war of all against all others) might be used to good effect in *Homo sapiens*'s quest to control disease causal agents. In 1928, it finally became known that the bacterial contents of certain forms of yeast molds battled and suppressed certain other forms of bacteria. One of the key figures in this discovery was the Scot, Alexander Fleming (1888–1955). After a long hiatus (potential paradigm shifts can take a long time to build up a head of steam before they take effect), Fleming's work was followed up by, among others, Ernst Chain, a refugee from Hitler's Germany.

In 1940, scientists tested their new antibiotic (killer bacteria) on caged lab mice which had been infected with streptococcal bacteria. Production difficulties (the yeast mold produced only minuscule quantities of penicillin) were finally overcome by American know-how (in Peoria, Illinois) and, by 1943, mass production had begun. In the event, penicillin was found to be wonderfully effective in suppressing a wide range of infections – among them septicemia, pneumonia and infections from abscessed teeth – which in former times had been major killers.

Given that the eventual breakthrough into penicillin had been a long, slow slog, we should also remind ourselves of the work in *chemistry*, in the early twentieth century, which had finally led to the application of *artificial* antibodies to dangerous disease conditions. In this, several key conceptual breakthroughs were made by Robert Koch's student and friend, Paul Ehrlich (1854–1915). Working in his laboratory in Frankfurt-am-Main, Ehrlich had come to realize that the human body's own immune system produced antibodies to combat invading disease agents; antibodies specific to a specific attacking disease agent were called *antitoxins*. Ehrlich's idea was that by injecting selected antitoxins (chemicals) into a person, the patient's own immune system would produce an increased number of antibodies to counter the disease agent: thus the patient would be cured.

Aside from Ehrlich (with his work on syphilis – in France, the disease phobia of the 1920s), three other students and associates of Koch made significant breakthroughs in the battle against what was a non-stigmatizing, but no less lethal disease – diphtheria. Reaching epidemic proportions by 1890 in the great cities of Europe and America, diphtheria was caused by a bacillus which manifested itself in a leathery blockage in the throat which produced a neurotoxin which generally killed its victims. Working at the end of that decade, Karl Fraenkel, Emil Behring and Shibasaburo Kitasato discovered that an attenuated form of the neurotoxin introduced into the bloodstream of a guinea pig led to the production of an antibody in the test animal which, in the form of serum (extracted from its blood), would induce immunity to diphtheria in a human being. Following on from this discovery, immunization campaigns were conducted among European and Euro-American school children. By 1940 (when the Second World War was already under way in Europe) diphtheria no longer counted as a major killer.

Yet, as the saying goes, "out of sight, out of mind." It would seem that a tax-paying public – which consisted of many Euro-Americans and Allied Europeans who were no friends of Germany – was loath to revise its (generally *unfavorable*) opinion of German-inspired medical science simply because it had caused one disease – diphtheria – to disappear. More had to be seen to be done. Aware of this perceptual barrier, medical scientists attempted to satisfy potential patrons and voters.

Coming out of long series of experiments in biochemistry were the *sulfa* drugs of the late 1930s and early 1940s. For a time they seemed to be effective against pneumonia, meningitis, polio, rheumatic fever, trachoma infections in the eye, mastoid infections in the ear and, to some degree, against tuberculosis. By this time, in Japan, TB had become a major killer even though (for reasons unknown to science) it had become less prevalent elsewhere in the West. Yet, despite the presence of sulfa drugs, well into the 1950s even in Great Britain, "heroic" treatments were still being applied to TB patients, including surgery to collapse part of an infected lung.

Other than its mixed bag of therapeutic breakthroughs and semi-breakthroughs, beginning in the mid-1960s, Western medicine began to be somewhat more successful in certain areas of surgery. It was about time. Three-quarters of a century earlier, private doctors in search of income (but who already knew something about pain killers) had begun to apply Joseph Lister's (1827–1912) insights about the need to sterilize the surgical instruments used for carving up well-heeled patients so they would not be infected by lethal germs and gangrene while still under the surgeon's care (and before they – or their heirs – had paid their bill – which usually ran into four or five figures).

By 1904 (when life expectancy at birth among rural Europeans and Americans was still not much more than 50) it had become common to recommend to middle-aged persons who no longer felt as peppy as they had while young that they submit to having a few meters of their intestines cut out (to remove what doctors told them were "blockages"). Among children it was becoming common to remove tonsils (seen as useless bits of flesh left over from some earlier stage of evolution from ape to man). We now know that tonsils are a useful part of the human immune system.

The first three-quarters of the twentieth century also witnessed the surgical removal of the cancerous breasts and under-arm lymph nodes of untold thousands of women, a procedure pioneered by William Halstead of Johns Hopkins Hospital. Not until the 1960s was Halstead's claim – that radical mastectomy removed all the cancer-causing agents in a patient's body – finally challenged by the Pittsburgh surgeon, Bernard Fisher. Belatedly in 1975, in an assessment of what had been achieved by all this cutting away of the flesh of fee-paying patients, the WHO announced that women who had submitted to heroic surgery were no more likely to be alive five years later than were women who had stoically let nature take its course – or gone off in search of a miraculous cure to Lourdes, the Roman Catholic shrine in southern France.

Nowadays, among mature adults and people over the age of 60, despite the more than US$20,000,000,000 spent on research since 1971, cancer continues to be a major killer. And among US surgeons working among the elderly insured, it continues to be a good source of income. It is unlikely these situations will change in the near future. Indeed, the US Cancer Institute predicts that among an increasingly aging US population, cancer incidence will double in the next few years. If current marketing trends continue, Western tobacco companies will meaningfully assist in realizing this prediction. Among women in the West as well as among the young of both sexes in the Non-west, tobacco sales are increasing. Thus – despite modern medicine – due to cultural pressures (TV ads and posters about how to be "youthful" and trendy) cancer continues to kill.

Less ambivalent is medicine's success in replacing used or damaged body parts. Beginning in 1960 surgeons in the UK devised a technique to replace hip joints which had worn down and left victims hardly able to walk. In the course of the next decade important improvements were made in techniques and materials: high grade plastic, for example, replaced squeaky stainless steel and screws. Yet, among active oldsters, the bone that surrounded the artificial implanted part often wore down, necessitating a second hip replacement job ten years or so after the first. Further research on this problem began at Cambridge University in 2001.

Beginning in the 1960s, and going well beyond the mere replacement of bits of bone by plastic, were the discoveries which permitted the removal of a defective major organ and its replacement by a similar organ from a "donor." The donor was very often a once healthy, young person of the same blood type who had just been killed in a car crash. However, in the case of kidneys – everyone is born with two, but can get along with just one – there is a worrisome trend for people in Non-western countries (such as prisoners in China) to "voluntarily" donate one of their kidneys for use in the West.

Making these organ transplants possible was the discovery of immuno-suppressive drugs (in 1951 cortisone and, since the late 1970s, cyclosporine). Otherwise, each human body tends to reject any organ grafted on to it that is taken from another human, or from the domesticated animal whose organs most closely resemble that of humans – the barnyard pig.

Beginning in 1967, heart transplants and open heart surgery began to be done with some regularity. Some of the patients who received this medical attention were still alive a year later.

Far more cost-efficient, in terms of prolonged life expectancy per unit of money sucked into the medical system, were the implanted pace-makers which regulated the number of heart-beats to keep them within a standard limit. It was not, however, clear that persons who were being kept artificially alive by a pace-maker remained mentally well-balanced.

Indeed, pace-makers or no, it has been reliably suggested that a quarter or more of the people living in the West in the year 2002 would, in the course of their adult careers, suffer from a serious mental condition. Though tens of thousands of adults have taken the drug *Prozac* (thought to be useful against depression), mental instability continues to be one of the great plagues confronting the West. And according to a recently published survey by the WHO, in those parts of the Non-west where chronic civil wars are raging and where economies are on the skids, more than a fifth of all infants are already exhibiting traits of mental illness. Specialists suggest that some of these disturbed infants may become the terrorists of the future.

Alternative medicine

Among many people living in the West whose income level permits them to pick and choose, high-tech high-cost biomedicine is not always their medicine of choice. This is particularly true of people who are suffering from the chronic ailments of old age – arthritis, rheumatism, failing diges-tion and the like – for which there is no simple biomedical treatment. But it is also true of the composite categories who identify either with one of the religious groupings who see biomedicine as the Devil's work, or with one of the New Age movements, with their stress on "holism" – mind and body as one.

Of particular importance to New Age people are what they take to be Chinese acupuncture procedures (which in fact have been decontextualized and made to be virtually unrecognizable in the land of their birth – see Chapter 6). Also important are what they take to be the ancient truths of Ayurvédic medicine (again, decontextualized and unrecognizable – see Chapter 5). Study of the culture of pharaonic Egypt is also infiltrated by people belonging to New Age movements (see Chapter 2).

The orthodox biomedical press tells us that 20 percent or more of the population in Britain – including educated middle-class persons – currently make some use of alternative medicine. In the US the figure is said to reach 40 percent. Similarly, in France, a high percentage of the population turn to alternative medicine to supplement biomedicine. This is thought to be their way of protesting against what the proud French claim is American domi-nation of everything that can be considered to be ultra-modern and new.

The oldest of the still surviving, coherent *secular* healing movements is known as *homeopathy*. Now officially recognized in Germany, France and the UK as a valid way to cure disease, the homeopathic movement was founded in Frankfurt-am-Main in 1796 by a dissident physician, Samuel Hahnemann. Troubled by the often terrible side-effects patients suffered when taking the conventional medicines used at the time (mercury and/or opium for example), Hahnemann built on the idea that nature (which is to say, the patient's own body) generated the brain impulses that caused the body to cure itself. Mind would take over and right whatever was wrong with body if it received the appropriate power of suggestion from an authority figure. The homeopathic practitioner assumes this role and has a patient ingest what she/he assures them is a proper cure (in fact it is merely water containing a tiny "trace" of a harmless drug). Mainstream press attacks on homeopathists simply serve to enhance their reputation among those categories of people who see bio-medicine as arrogant and avaricious.

In the US today no one is allowed to forget that the US Public Health Service conducted experiments on African-Americans suffering from syphilis in a hospital in Tuskegee, Alabama between 1932 and 1972. During these 40 years, minority-group patients were given to understand that they were all being treated with modern, approved drugs (first with Ehrlich's Salvarsan, then with updated cures). However, what was in fact happening was that half the patients were being given placebos (injections containing no medicine). Public Health Authority doctors claimed that this procedure would permit them to study the full long-term degenerative effects of syphilis on the nervous system. In the event none of their findings were of any scientific merit.

Similarly, no one today is permitted to forget that German medical doctors performed all manner of deadly experiments on gypsies, Slavs, Jews and homosexuals incarcerated in Hitler's concentration camps between the years 1939 and 1945. Neither are we allowed to forget that during those same years, Japanese physicians also carried out all sorts of experiments (induced bubonic plague, cholera, syphilis, etc.) on prisoners of war (both Asian and European). In German medical schools today, as a partial corrective on the terrible policies of half a century ago, courses in the history of medicine deliberately focus students' attention on the evolution of medical ethics. Perhaps more should be done in this area in the US.

Biomedicine in the Non-west c. 2002

At the beginning of this chapter we found that in the years since 1940 modern Western medicine has acquired the *ability* to cure a wide range of heretofore intractable diseases. Going beyond this, Western science (exemplified by the human genome project and what follows on from it) promises that more diseases and more unpleasant conditions – especially those that are genetically related and come on with old age – will eventually be brought under control, provided of course that adequate funding is forthcoming. But as we have also seen, 85 percent of the people alive at the present time (fellow human beings generally, but not always, living in the Non-west) do not have the financial resources needed to make use of even a tiny fraction of the services that biomedicine can, in theory, provide. This is exemplified in case-specific situations.

Paul Farmer, the Harvard anthropologist and practicing medical doctor, has brilliantly demonstrated with reference to named poor persons in Peru and in Haiti (formerly called Hispaniola: Chapter 7), that these people would jump at the chance to have access to the full battery of Western drugs needed to control their HIV condition. They would also jump at the chance to use the modern range of drugs needed to control the tuberculosis (now often in drug-resistant form) which is the opportunistic killer that so frequently attacks HIV/AIDS victims.

However, in most parts of the world, for reasons associated with the "legitimate" returns due to investors and the well-deserved sums paid to boards of directors (each annual salary usually amounting to US$500,000 or more) the requisite drugs simply are not to be found. Even if they were by some miracle made to be physically present through the benevolence of a Western pharmaceutical company (and sold at costs calculated to preserve a fair return on the company's "intellectual property rights"), they would still remain completely out of range of ordinary cash-strapped people. The current cost of the treatment complex which stabilizes the HIV/AIDS condition of a person living in the West (who is covered by insurance) is around $50,000 a year. This is over 150 times more than the sum that chronically poor individuals in the Non-west have for all their yearly requirements – food, clothing, shelter, school fees and the rest.

In the case of South Africa – the non-white country which at the moment is most at threat from AIDS because of earlier and current employment patterns – this means that more than one in four of the young people now aged 15 or less can expect to die of AIDS. It also means that nearly half the babies being born will be orphans, easy prey for the Fagins of the world.

To its credit, in September 2002 the post-apartheid South African government sponsored a "sanitation" awareness conference which was attended by 104 of the world's heads of government. However, because the absent head of the world's most powerful nation let it be known that "sanitation" was of secondary importance compared to the needs of development as defined by the IMF, very little was achieved. Some historians at the time realized that this statement was almost identical to that made by the Raj (the Government of India) in 1889 when countering Florence Nightingale's claim that unsanitary conditions were undermining the health of rural populations (see pages 123–4).

Indeed, the health situation in post-Raj, post-Independence India continues to be dire. If Government indifference to the health of its people – one-quarter of humanity – as currently exemplified by its responses to malaria, to TB and to communal violence in Gujarat – continues unchanged, it is likely that the country's HIV/AIDS epidemic (which as of the year 2001 had already established a foothold) will run rampant and destroy nearly the entire generation of educated young people on which the future of the sub-continent depends. It will also destroy the lives of many young medical doctors (educated at the expense of Indian taxpayers) who had planned to migrate to London, Manchester and other cities in the island kingdom to staff chronically undermanned hospitals and clinics.

In Uganda (East Africa), the destruction of nearly an entire generation by HIV/AIDS and attendant opportunistic diseases has already happened. However, the situation there has finally been stabilized by firm government action – a mass education campaign about the merits of condoms for safe sex. Yet, despite their huge potential in preventing infectious diseases, sex-education programs for at-risk youthful populations remain controversial almost everywhere, except in the Netherlands and the Scandinavian countries.

As in Uganda and South Africa, HIV/AIDS has also become a major killer in the Russian Federation – a country (under its old name, the USSR) which before 1989 was counted among the developed nations of the world. Now, however, (less than a quarter of a century after the promises offered at Alma Ata in 1978), life expectancy at birth of the ordinary Russian *male* has dropped ten years. This massive decline (unparalleled among Caucasian civilians since the end of the Second World War) has been brought about by the collapse of state-provided medical facilities under pressure from the IMF. These phenomena have been accompanied by a massive increase in rates of smoking (lung cancer) and of alcohol use (heart and liver problems), and of violence and suicide brought on by despair.

Conclusion

As a medical historian quoted by Paul Farmer (of Harvard) put it in 1997:

> The last half-century has seen the triumphant emergence of medicine as a fully scientific discipline of proven effectiveness in curing and preventing life-threatening diseases. Yet it has also seen the emergence of a widening gap in the provisioning (and non-provisioning) of effective health services for the privileged few and the underprivileged many.

Since that was written, great quantities of information published by the WHO, the European journal *Tropical Medicine and International Health* and the *American Journal of Tropical Medicine and Hygiene* further confirms that it is *fallacious* to hold that Non-western peoples would reject Western bio-medicine, if it were made available to them, in favor of "traditional" Ayurvédic, Unani Tibb, systems of Systematic Correspondences, Voodoo, Pre-Columbian, or whatever other type of pre-scientific medicine their distant ancestors may once have used.

As we saw in Chapter 1 (page 9) medical anthropologists and medico-cultural historians now recognize that there never was, in any corner of the globe, any such thing as a "traditional culture" unchanged from "time immemorial." Instead, in each society, each upcoming generation has reassessed the wisdom they received from their elders, keeping that bit which they saw as useful, and rejecting the rest.

The re-emergence of the Orientalist "unchanged since time immemorial" argument among non-reflexive Westerners when discussing Non-western peoples' health situations suggests a regression to the conceptual world illustrated at the microscopic level by Alexander Fleming-style bacteria, engaged in their war of one against all. It is to be hoped that open-minded study and re-assessment of medical and disease history in changing cultural settings will enable Westerners to see this Orientalist conceit for what it is and to send it off to the Museum of Obsolete Ideas.

In 1876, the year in which Robert Koch first brought modern medicine into being in his backyard lab, the prototype postmodern philosopher of mental well-being stated: "We cannot be fully self-realized [or happy] so long as everything around us suffers and creates suffering. . . . We cannot be moral so long as the course of human affairs is determined by force, deception and injustice." As historians of medicine and of disease we are aware of what needs to be done. The future remains open.

Further reading

Paul Farmer, *Infections and Inequalities: the modern plagues* (updated edition) (University of California Press, 1999) (with powerfully stated end-notes, esp. p. 316). Richard Guerrant, "Why America Must Care about Tropical Medicine: threats to global health and security from tropical infectious diseases" (Presidential Address given before the American Society of Tropical Medicine and Hygiene, 9 December 1997) *American Journal of Tropical Medicine and Hygiene* 59 (1), (1998), 3–16. Roy Porter, last six chapters in his *The Greatest Benefit to Mankind: a medical history* (HarperCollins, 1997) with massive bibliography. Sheldon Watts, last chapter in his *Epidemics and History: disease, power and imperialism* (London: Yale, 1997); contains extensive end-note references.

Bibliography

Basic journals in the history of medicine

Bulletin of the History of Medicine, Baltimore, Johns Hopkins University Press.
Journal of the History of Medicine and Allied Sciences, Farmington, CT: University of Connecticut.
Journal of World History, Honolulu, University of Hawai'i Press.
Medical History, London, England: Wellcome Institute for the History of Medicine.
Social History of Medicine, Oxford: Oxford University Press.

Preface

Bentley, Jerry H. (1996) "Shapes of World History in Twentieth Century Scholarship" in Michael Adas (ed.) *Essays on Global and Comparative History*, Washington, DC: American Historical Association.
Chakrabarty, Dipesh (2000) *Provincializing Europe: postcolonial thought and historical difference*, Princeton, NJ: Princeton University Press.
Goody, Jack (1996) *The East in the West*, Cambridge: Cambridge University Press.
Said, Edward (1978) *Orientalism: Western conceptions of the Orient*, London: Routledge and Kegan Paul. The pioneering conceptualization of The Other.
Segal, Daniel (2000) " 'Western Civ' and the Staging of History in American Higher Education," *American Historical Review* 105 (3): 770–803.
Stokes, Gale (2001) "The Fates of Human Societies: a review of recent macro-histories," *American Historical Review* 106 (2): 508–25.

I Sickness and health, a global concern

Bates, Don (ed.) (1995) *Knowledge and Scholarly Medical Traditions*, New York: Cambridge University Press.
Bynum, William and Roy Porter (eds) (1993) *Companion Encyclopedia of the History of Medicine*, London: Routledge.
Creaton, Heather (1990) "Starting Research in Medical History: preparing the ground," *Society for the History of Medicine* 3: 285–9.
Cunningham, Andrew and Perry Williams (eds) (1992) *The Laboratory Revolution in Medicine*, Cambridge: Cambridge University Press.

Diamond, Jared (1997) *Guns, Germs, and Steel: the fates of human societies*, New York: W. W. Norton and Co.

Ewald, Paul W. (1994) *The Evolution of Infectious Disease*, New York: Oxford University Press. Musings by a biological theorist.

Evans-Pritchard, E. E. (1937) *Witchcraft, Oracles and Magic Among the Azande*, Oxford: Clarendon Press.

Feierman, Steven and John Janzen (eds) (1992) *The Social Basis of Health and Healing in Africa*, Berkeley, University of California Press.

Flannery, Tim (2000) *The Eternal Frontier: an ecological history of North America and its people*, London: Heinemann.

French, Roger (1994) "Astrology in Medical Practice," in Luis García Ballester, Roger French, Jon Arrizabalaga and Andrew Cunningham (eds) *Practical Medicine from Salerno to the Black Death*, New York: Cambridge University Press.

Gentilcore, David (1998) *Healers and Healing in Early Modern Italy*, Manchester: Manchester University Press.

Helvoort, Ton van (1994) "History of Virus Research in the Twentieth Century: the problem of conceptual continuity," *History of Science* 32: 185–224.

Kiple, Kenneth (1993) *The Cambridge World History of Human Disease*, Cambridge: Cambridge University Press. To be used with caution.

MacLeod, Roy and Donald Denoon (eds) (1991) *Health and Healing in Tropical Australia and Papua New Guinea*, Townsville, Australia: James Cook University.

McNeill, William M. (1976) *Plagues and Peoples*, London: Penguin. The pioneering work.

Nielsen, Richard (2001) "The Kensington Runestone," *Scandinavian Studies* 72 (1). Finally authenticating the Norse presence.

Pomata, Gianna (1998) *Contracting a Cure: patients, healers and law in early modern Bologna*, Baltimore: Johns Hopkins University Press.

Porter, Roy and Andrew Wear (eds) (1987) *Problems and Methods in the History of Medicine*, London: Croom Helm.

Rosenberg, Charles E. (1989) "Disease in History: frames and framers," *Milbank Quarterly* 67 (supplement 1): 1–15.

Vaughan, Megan (1994) "Healing and Curing: issues in the social history and anthropology of medicine in Africa," *Social History of Medicine* 7: 283–95.

Watts, Sheldon (1984) *A Social History of Western Europe, 1450–1720: tensions and solidarities among rural people*, London: Hutchinson University Library.

Watts, Sheldon (2001) "Yellow Fever Immunities in West Africa and the Americas in the Age of Slavery and Beyond: a reappraisal," *Journal of Social History* 34 (4): 955–68, 975–6.

Woodward, John and Robert Jütte (eds) (1996) *Coping with Sickness: perspectives on health care, past and present*, Sheffield, England: European Association for the History of Medicine and Health Publications.

Wright, Peter and Andrew Treacher (1982) *The Problem of Medical Knowledge: examining the social construction of medicine*, Edinburgh: Edinburgh University Press.

2 Pharaonic Egypt and the pre-conquest New World

Alchon, Suzanne (1991) *Native Society and Disease in Colonial Ecuador*, Cambridge: Cambridge University Press.

Allen, Robert (1997) "Agriculture and the Origins of the State in Ancient Egypt," *Explorations in Economic History* 34: 135–54. Discusses implications of low population densities, non-urbanization, the impact of geography and the slow transition from foraging to agriculture.

Bastien, Joseph (1987) *Healers of the Andes: Kallawaya herbalists and their medicinal plants*, Salt Lake City: University of Utah Press.

Bastien, Joseph and John Donahue (eds) (1981) *Health in the Andes*, New York: American Anthropological Association.

Burke, Paul F. (1996) "Malaria in the Greco-Roman World: a historical and epidemiological survey," in Wolfgand Haase (ed.) *Aufstieg und Niedergang der römischen Weld Teil II*, Band 37, Berlin: de Gruyter.

Cann, Rebecca L. (2001) "Genetic Clues to Dispersal in Human Populations: retracing the past from the present," *Science* 291: 1742–8.

Clendinnen, Inga (1985) "The Cost of Courage in Aztec Society," *Past and Present* 107: 44–89.

Davies, W. V. and R. Walker (1993) *Biological Anthropology and the Study of Ancient Egypt*, London: British Museum Press.

Dobyns, Henry F. (1989) "More Methodological Perspectives on Historical Demography," *Ethnohistory* 36 (3): 288–9.

Estes, J. W. (1993) *The Medical Skills of Ancient Egypt*, Canton, MA: Science History Publications.

Fagan, Brian (1984) *The Aztecs*, New York: W. H. Freeman and Co.

Grmeck, Mirko (1989) *Diseases in the Ancient Greek World*, Baltimore: Johns Hopkins University Press.

Kidwell, Clara Sue (1982) "Aztec and European Medicine in the New World, 1521–1600," in Lola Romanucci-Ross, D. Moerman and L. Tancredi (eds) *The Anthropology of Medicine: from culture to method*, New York: Praeger/J. F. Bergin.

Martin, Simon and Nikolai Grube (2000) *Chronicle of the Maya Kings and Queens*, London: Thames and Hudson. Contains recent research findings on the civilization as a whole.

Meeks, Dimitri and Christine Favard-Meeks (1997) *Daily Life of the Egyptian Gods*, London: John Murray.

Nunn, John F. D. (1996) *Ancient Egyptian Medicine*, London: British Museum Press.

Nunn, John (2000) "Disease," in Donald Redford (ed.) *Oxford Encyclopedia of Ancient Egypt*, New York: Oxford University Press.

Nunn, John and E. Tapp (2000) "Tropical Diseases in Ancient Egypt," *Transactions of the Royal Society of Tropical Medicine and Hygiene* 94: 147–53.

Ortiz de Montellano, Bernard R. (1990) *Aztec Medicine, Health and Nutrition*, New Brunswick, NJ: Rutgers University Press.

Palter, Robert (1993) "Black Athena, Afro-centrism, and the History of Science," *History of Science* 31: 263–87. An assessment of the impact, or non-impact, of Egyptian medicine on Greek medicine in Alexandria.

Redford, Donald (ed.) (2000) *Oxford Encyclopedia of Ancient Egypt*, New York: Oxford University Press.

Ritner, Robert K. (2000) "Magic in Medicine," in Donald Redford (ed.) *Oxford Encyclopedia of Ancient Egypt*, New York: Oxford University Press.

Ross, Ronald (1910) "Missionaries and the Campaign against Malaria," *Journal of Tropical Medicine and Hygiene* 13: 183.

Ubelaker, Douglas H. (1992) "Patterns of Demographic Change," in John W. Verano and D. Ubelaker (eds) *Disease and Demography in the Americas*, Washington, DC: The Smithsonian Institution Press.

3 Pluralism in ancient Greece

Edelstein, Ludwig (1967) *Ancient Medicine*, Baltimore: Johns Hopkins University Press.

Lloyd, G. E. R. (1982) *Science, Folklore and Ideology: studies in the life sciences in ancient Greece*, Cambridge: Cambridge University Press. Stresses the multiplicity of notions about reality and the importance of open debate in ancient Greece.

Lloyd, G. E. (1990) *Methods and Problems in Greek Science*, Cambridge University Press.

Lloyd, G. E. (1992) "The Transformations of Ancient Medicine," *Bulletin of the History of Medicine* 66 (1): Spring.

Longrigg, James (1992) "Epidemic, Ideas and Classical Athenian Society," in Terence Ranger and Paul Slack (eds) *Epidemics and Ideas: essays on the historical perception of pestilence*, Cambridge: Cambridge University Press.

Nutton, Vivian (1983) "The Seeds of Disease: an explanation of contagion and infection from the Greeks to the Renaissance," *Medical History* 27: 1–34.

Nutton, Vivian (1993) "Humoralism," in William Bynum and Roy Porter (eds) *Companion Encyclopedia of the History of Medicine*, London: Routledge.

von Staden, Heinrich (1989) *Herophilus: the art of medicine in early Alexandria*, Cambridge: Cambridge University Press.

4 Evolution of medical systems in the Middle East

Abu-Lugard, Janet (1989) *Before European Hegemony: the world system A.D. 1250–1350*, New York: Oxford University Press.

Conrad, Lawrence (1992) "Epidemic Disease in Formal and Popular Thought in Early Islamic Society," in Terence Ranger and Paul Slack (eds) *Epidemics and Ideas: essays on the historical perception of pestilence*, Cambridge: Cambridge University Press.

Conrad, Lawrence (1993) "Arab-Islamic Medicine," in William Bynum and Roy Porter (eds) *Companion Encyclopedia of the History of Medicine*, London: Routledge.

Conrad, Lawrence (1995) "The Arab-Islamic Medical Tradition," in L. Conrad, M. Neve, V. Nutton, R. Porter and A. Wear (eds) *The Western Medical Tradition 800 BC to AD 1800*, Cambridge: Cambridge University Press.

Dols, Michael (1977) *The Black Death in the Middle East*, Princeton NJ: Princeton University Press.

Dols, Michael (1987) "The Origins of the Islamic Hospital: myth and reality," *Bulletin of the History of Medicine and Allied Sciences* 61: 367–90.

Dols, Michael (1992) Diana Immisch (ed.) *Majnun: the madman in medieval Islamic society*, Oxford: Clarendon Press.

Gamal, Adil (ed.), Michael Dols (trans.) (1984) *Medieval Islamic Medicine: Ibn Ridwan's Treatise "On the Prevention of Bodily Ills in Egypt"*, Berkeley: University of California Press.

Goitein, S. D. (1971) *A Mediterranean Society: the Jewish communities of the Arab world as portrayed in the documents of the Cairo Geniza*, Vol II, *The Community*, Berkeley: University of California Press.

Hourani, Albert (1991) *A History of the Arab Peoples*, London: Faber and Faber. An excellent introduction.

Huff, Toby (1993) *The Rise of Early Modern Science: Islam, China and the West*, Cambridge: Cambridge University Press. Suspect: exemplifies the Eurocentric, learned approach.

Jacquart, Danielle and Françoise Micheau (1996) *La Médecine Arabe et l'Occident Médiéval*, Paris: Editions Maisonneuve et Larose.

Johnstone, Penelope (trans.) (1998) *Ibn Qayyim al-Jawziyya Medicine of the Prophet*, Leiden: The Islamic Texts Society.

Leiser, Gary (1983) "Medical Education in Islamic Lands from the Seventh to the Fourteenth Century," *Journal of the History of Medicine and Allied Sciences* 38: 48–75.

Meyerhof, Max (1984) "Thirty-three Clinical Observations by Rhazes (circa 900 AD)," in Penelope Johnstone (ed.) *Studies in Medieval Arabic Medicine: theory and practice*, London: Variorum Reprints.

Siraisi, Nancy (1987) *Avicenna in Renaissance Italy: the Canon and medical teaching in Italian universities after 1500*, Princeton, NJ: Princeton University Press.

5 Health and disease in India before 1869

Basham, A. L. (1976) "The Practice of Medicine in Ancient and Medieval India," in Charles Leslie (ed.) *Asian Medical Systems: a comparative study*, Berkeley, CA: University of California Press.

Breckenridge, Carol A. and Peter van der Veer (eds) (1993) *Orientalism and the Postcolonial Predicament: perspectives on South Asia*, Philadelphia: University of Pennsylvania Press.

Caldwell, J. C., P. H. Reddy and Pat Caldwell, "The Social Component of Mortality Decline: an investigation of South India employing alternative methodologies," *Population Studies* 37: 185–205. Largely anthropological, containing suggestive hints about pre-colonial concepts and practices.

Durkin-Longley, Maureen (1982) "Ayurveda in Nepal: a medical belief system in action," unpublished thesis, University of Wisconsin-Madison. Chapter 1, background.

Gupta, Brahamananda (1976) "Indigenous Medicine in 19th and 20th century Bengal," in C. M. Leslie (ed.) *Asian Medical Systems: a comparative study*, Berkeley: University of California Press.

Jaggi, O. P. (1977) *History of Science, Technology and Medicine in India*, Vol. 8, *Medicine in Medieval India*, Delhi: Atma Ram & Sons. Heavily tainted by Raj categories, but this and other volumes contain some useful information not easy to access elsewhere.

Khare, R. S. (1963) "Folk Medicine in a North Indian Village," *Human Organization* 22 (1): 36–40. Anthropological.

Nicholas, Ralph W. (1981) "The Goddess Sitala and Epidemic Smallpox in Bengal," *Journal of Asian Studies* 41 (1): 21–44.

Sharma, Kailish (1986) "Ayurvedic Medicine: past and present," in Teizo Ogawa (ed.) *History of Traditional Medicine*, Susuno-shi, Shizuoka, Japan: The Taniquchi Foundation.

Subrahmanyam, Sanjay (2001) *Penumbral Visions: making polities in early modern South India*, Ann Arbor, MI: University of Michigan Press. A nail in the coffin of the India "unchanged since time immemorial" thesis.

Talbot, Cynthia (2001) *Precolonial India in Practice: society, religion and identity in medieval Andhra*, Oxford: Oxford University Press. Demonstrates the vibrant nature of medieval society around Hyderabad: overturns the "unchanged since time immemorial" thesis.

Wujastyk, Dominik (1993) "Indian Medicine," in William Bynum and Roy Porter (eds) *Companion Encyclopedia of the History of Medicine*, London: Routledge.

Zimmermann, Francis (1987) *The Jungle and the Aroma of Meats: an ecological theme in Hindu medicine*, Berkeley: University of California Press.

Zimmermann, Francis (1989) "Terminological Problems in the Process of Editing and Translating Sanskrit Medical Texts," in Paul U. Unschuld (ed.) *Approaches to Traditional Chinese Medical Literature*, Amsterdam: Kluwer Academic Publishers.

Zimmermann, Francis (1995) "The Scholar, the Wise Man, and Universals: three aspects of Ayurvedic medicine," in Don Bates (ed.) *Knowledge and the Scholarly Medical Traditions*, Cambridge: Cambridge University Press.

Zysk, K. G. (1991) *Asceticism and Healing in Ancient India: medicine in the Buddhist monastery*, New York: Oxford University Press.

6 Medicine and disease in China to 1840

Bray, Francesca (1993) "Chinese Medicine," in William Bynum and Roy Porter (eds) *Companion Encyclopedia of the History of Medicine*, London: Routledge.

Bray, Francesca (1997) *Technology and Gender: fabrics of power in late imperial China*, Berkeley: University of California Press.

Bray, Francesca (1999) "Chinese Health Beliefs," in John R. Hinnells and Roy Porter (eds) *Religion, Health and Suffering*, London: Kegan Paul International.

Cooper, William C. and Nathan Sivin (1973) "Man as a Medicine: pharmacological and ritual aspects of traditional therapy using drugs derived from the human body," in Shigeru Nakayama and Nathan Sivin (eds) *Chinese Science*, Cambridge, MA: The MIT Press.

Cullen, Christopher (1993) "Patients and Healers in Late Imperial China: evidence from the Jinpingmei," *History of Science* 31: 99–150.

Epler, D. C. (1980) "Bloodletting in Early Chinese Medicine and its Relation to the Origin of Acupuncture," *Bulletin of the History of Medicine and Allied Sciences* 54: 337–67.

Epler, D. C. (1988) "The Concept of Disease in an Ancient Chinese Medical Text: the discourse on cold-damage disorders (Shang-han Lun)," *Journal of the History of Medicine and Allied Sciences* 43: 8–35.

Furth, Charlotte (1999) *A Flourishing Yin: medicine and gender in Late Imperial China*, Berkeley: University of California Press.

Grant, Joanna (1998) "Medical Practice in the Ming Dynasty: a practitioner's view: evidence from Wang ji's shishan yi'an," *Chinese Science* 15: 37–80.

Hart, Roger (1999) "Beyond Science and Civilization: a post-Needham critique," *East Asian Science, Technology and Medicine* 16: 88–114.

Hymens, Robert (1987) "Not Quite Gentlemen: physicians in the Sung and Yuan," *Chinese Science* 8: 9–76.

Kaptchuk, Ted (1983) *The Web that Has No Weaver: understanding Chinese medicine*, New York: Congdon and Weed.

Kleinman, Arthur (1980) *Patients and Healers in the Context of Culture: an exploration of the borderline between anthropology, medicine and psychiatry*, Berkeley: University of California Press.

Kuriyama, Shigehisa (1994) "The Imagination of Winds and the Development of the Chinese Conception of the Body," in Angela Zito and Tani Barlow (eds) *Body, Subject & Power in China*, Chicago: University of Chicago Press.

Kuriyama, Shigehisa (1995) "Visual Knowledge in Classical Chinese Medicine," in Don Bates (ed.) *Knowledge and the Scholarly Medical Traditions*, Cambridge: Cambridge University Press.

Kuriyama, Shigehisa (1999) *The Expressiveness of the Body and the Divergence of Greek and Chinese Medicine*, New York: Zone Books.

Leslie, Charles and Allan Young (1992) *Paths to Asian Medical Knowledge*, Berkeley: University of California Press.

Lloyd, Geoffrey and Nathan Silvin (2002) *The Way and the Word: science and medicine in early China and Greece*, London: Yale.

Lu Gwei-Djen and Joseph Needham (1980) *Celestial Lancets: a history and rationale of acupuncture and moxa*, Cambridge: Cambridge University Press. Findings much modified by more recent research.

Needham, Joseph with Lu Gwei-djin (1966) "Medicine and Chinese Culture: clerks and craftsmen in China and the West," in Mansel Davies (1990) *A Selection from the Writings of Joseph Needham*, Sussex, England: The Book Guild Ltd. Needham was the English-language pioneer in the study of Chinese science. The questions he posed remain valid; some of his answers have been sent to the Museum of the Obsolete.

Pomeranz, Kenneth (2000) *The Great Divergence: China, Europe and the making of the modern world economy*, Princeton, NJ: Princeton University Press.

Porkert, Manfried (1974) *The Theoretical Foundations of Chinese Medicine: systems of correspondence*, Cambridge, MA: MIT. A pioneering European-language work of some value to historians.

Sivin, Nathan (1988) "Science and Medicine in Imperial China – the state of the field," *The Journal of Asian Studies* 47 (1): 41-90 (includes 17 pp of bibliography).

Sivin, Nathan (1995) "Text and Experience in Classical Chinese Medicine: in Don Bates (ed.) *Knowledge and the Scholarly Medical Traditions*, Cambridge: Cambridge University Press.

Sivin, Nathan (1995) *Medicine, Philosophy and Religion in Ancient China: researches and reflections*, Aldershot, UK: Variorum.

Unshuld, Paul U. (1985) (translated from the German by Susan Mango and Charles Leslie) *Medicine in China: a history of ideas*, Berkeley: University of California Press.

Unshuld, Paul U. (1998) (trans. by Nigel Wiseman) *Chinese Medicine*, Brookline, MA: Paradigm Publications. A brief introduction.

Wang, Jen-Yi (1991) "Psychosomatic Illness in the Chinese Cultural Context," in Lola Romanucci-Ross, D. Moerman and L. Tancredi (eds) *The Anthropology of Medicine: from culture to method*, New York: Bergin & Garvey.

Wong, R. Bin (1997) *China Transformed: historical change and the limits of European experience*, Ithaca, NY: Cornell University Press.

7 The globalization of disease after 1450

Alchon, Suzanne Austin (1991) *Native Society and Disease in Colonial Ecuador*, Cambridge: Cambridge University Press.

Baker, Brenda J. and George J. Armelagos (1988) "The Origin and Antiquity of Syphilis: paleopathologic diagnosis and interpretation," *Current Anthropology* 29 (5): 732–7.

Bastien, Joseph W. (ed.) (1985) *Health in the Andes*, New York: American Anthropological Association.

Black, F. L. (1994) "An Explanation of High Death Rates among New World Peoples When in Contact with Old World Diseases," *Perspectives in Biology and Medicine* 37 (2), 292–307.

Blackburn, Robin (1997) *The Making of New World Slavery: from the Baroque to the modern 1492–1800*, London: Verso.

Braudel, Fernand (1985) *Civilization & Capitalism, 15th–18th Century*, Vol. 3, *The Perspective of the World*, London: Collins/Fontana Press.

Cook, Noble David and W. George Lovell (eds) (1991) *"Secret Judgments of God": Old World disease in colonial Spanish America*, Norman, OK: University of Oklahoma Press.

Cook, Noble David (1998) *Born to Die: disease and New World conquest, 1492–1650*, Cambridge: Cambridge University Press.

Crosby, Alfred W. (1972) *The Columbian Exchange: biological consequences of 1492*, Westport, CT: Greenwood Press. A pioneering work: some of its core concepts are now museum pieces.

Geary, Patrick (2002) *The Myth of Nations: the medieval origins of Europe*, Princeton, NJ: Princeton University Press. On the diverse origins of the settler/inhabitants of post-Roman Empire Europe.

Gruzinski, Serge (1993) *The Conquest of Mexico: the incorporation of Indian societies in the Western world, 16th–18th centuries*, Cambridge: Cambridge University Press.

Hall, Richard (1998) *Empires of the Monsoon: a history of the Indian Ocean and its invaders*, London: HarperCollins.

Henige, David (1986) "When did Smallpox reach the New World (and why does it matter)?" in Paul Lovejoy (ed.) *Africans in Bondage: studies in slavery and the slave trade*, Madison: University of Wisconsin Press: 11–26.

Inikori, Joseph and Stanley L. Engerman (eds) (1992) *The Atlantic Slave Trade: effects on economies, societies, and peoples in Africa, the Americas and Europe*, Durham, NC: University of North Carolina Press.

Joralemon, Donald (1982) "New World Depopulation and the Case of Disease," *Journal of Anthropological Research* 38: 109–27.

McCaa, Robert (1995) "Spanish and Nahuatl Views on Smallpox and Demographic Catastrophe in Mexico," *Journal of Interdisciplinary History* 25: 397–431.

MacLeod, D. Peter (1992) "Microbes and Muskets: smallpox and the participation of the Amerindian allies of New France in the Seven Years War," *Ethnohistory* 30 (1): 42–64.

MacLeod, Roy and Milton Lewis (eds) (1988) *Disease, Medicine, and Empire: perspectives on western medicine and the experience of European expansion*, London: Routledge.

Miller, Joseph (1988) *Way of Death: merchant capitalism and the Angolan slave trade, 1730–1830*, London: James Currey.

Pomeranz, Kenneth (2000) *The Great Divergence: China, Europe and the making of the modern world economy*, Princeton, NJ: Princeton University Press.

Porter, H. C. (1979) *The Inconstant Savage: England and the North American Indian 1500–1660*, London: Duckworth.

Stannard, David E. (1992) *American Holocaust: Columbus and the conquest of the New World*, Oxford: Oxford University Press.

Thomas, Hugh (1993) *Conquest: Montezuma, Cortés, and the fall of Old Mexico*, New York, Simon & Schuster.

Thomas, Hugh (1998) *The Slave Trade: the history of the Atlantic slave trade 1440–1870*, London: Papermac.

Thornton, John (1992) *Africa and Africans in the Making of the Atlantic World*, Cambridge: Cambridge University Press.

Ubelaker, Douglas H. (1992) "Patterns of Demographic Change in the Americas," *Human Biology* 64 (3): 361–79.

Verano, John W. and Douglas H. Ubelaker (eds) (1992) *Disease and Demography in the Americas*, Washington, DC: Smithsonian Institution Press.

Watts, Sheldon (1997) "Smallpox in the New World and in the Old: from holocaust to eradication, 1518–1977," in *Epidemics and History: disease, power and imperialism*, London: Yale University Press.

Wong, R. Bin (2002) "The Search for European Differences and Domination in the Early Modern World: a view from Asia," *The American Historical Review* 107 (2) April: 447–69.

Wright, Richard (1993) *Stolen Continents: the Indian story*, London: Pimlico.

8 Medicine and disease in the West, 1050–1840

Cook, Harold (1990) "The New Philosophy and Medicine in Seventeenth Century England," in D. C. Lindberg and R. S. Westman (eds) *Reappraisals of the Scientific Revolution*, Cambridge: Cambridge University Press.

Cooter, Roger, M. Harrison and S. Sturdy (eds) (1999) *Medicine and Modern Warfare*, Amsterdam/Atlanta, GA: Rodopi.

Debus, Allen (1991) *The French Paracelsians*, Cambridge: Cambridge University Press.

Grell, Ole Peter (ed.) (1998) *Paracelsus: the man and his reputation, his ideas and their transformation*, Leiden: Brill.

Maddicott, J. R. (1997) "Plague in Seventh-Century England," *Past and Present* 156: 7–54.

Murphy, Terence (1979) "The French Medical Profession's Perception of its Social Function between 1776 and 1830," *Medical History* 23: 259–78.

Nagy, Doreen (1988) *Popular Medicine in 17th Century England*, Bowling Green, OH: Bowling Green State University Popular Press.

Park, Katharine (1992) "Medicine and society in Medieval Europe, 500–1500," in Andrew Wear (ed.) *Medicine in Society: historical essays*, Cambridge: Cambridge University Press.

Porter, Dorothy and Roy Porter (1989) *Patients' Progress: doctors and doctoring in eighteenth-century England*, Stanford, CA: Stanford University Press.

Porter, Roy (1989) "The Language of Quackery in England, 1660–1800," in Peter Burke and Roy Porter (eds) *The Social History of Language*, Cambridge: Cambridge University Press.

Porter, Roy (1992) (ed.) *The Popularization of Medicine, 1650-1850*, London: Routledge.

Porter, Roy (1997) *The Greatest Benefit to Mankind*, Chapters 5, 8, 9, 10 and their bibliographic references. London: HarperCollins Publishers.

Ramsey, Matthew (1992) "The Popularization of Medicine in France, 1650–1900," in Roy Porter (ed.) *The Popularization of Medicine, 1650–1850*, London: Routledge.

Siraisi, Nancy (1990) *Medieval & Early Renaissance Medicine: an introduction to knowledge and practice*, Chicago, IL: University of Chicago Press.

Watts, Sheldon (1997) *Epidemics and History: disease, power and imperialism*, Chapters 1 (Plague); 2 (Leprosy); 4 (Syphilis); and bibliographic references. London: Yale University Press.

Wear, Andrew (1989) "Medical Practice and Late Seventeenth- and Early Eighteenth-century England: continuity and union," in Roger French and Andrew Wear (eds) *The Medical Revolution of the Seventeenth Century*, Cambridge: Cambridge University Press.

9 The birth of modern scientific medicine

Barnes, Barry (1990) "Sociological Theories of Scientific Knowledge", in R. C. Olby, G. N. Cantor, J. R. R. Christie and M. J. S. Hodge (eds) *Companion to the History of Modern Science*, London: Routledge.

Bell, Frances and Robert Millward (1998) "Public Health Expenditure and Mortality in England and Wales, 1870–1914," *Continuity and Change* 13 (2): 221–49.

Bellamy, Christine (1988) *Administration: centre-local relations, 1871–1919*, Manchester: Manchester University Press.

Bonner, Thomas N. (1995) *Becoming a Physician: medical education in Britain, France, Germany and the United States, 1750–1945*, Oxford: Oxford University Press.

Bracegirdle, Brian (1993) "The Microscopical Tradition," in W. Bynum and R. Porter (eds) *Companion Encyclopedia of the History of Medicine*, London: Routledge.

Brock, T. D. (1988) *Robert Koch: a life in medicine and bacteriology*, Madison, WN: University of Wisconsin Press.

Broman, Thomas (1995) *The Transformation of German Academic Medicine, 1750–1820*, Cambridge: Cambridge University Press.

Brundage, Anthony (1988) *England's "Prussian Minister," Edwin Chadwick and the Politics of Government Growth, 1832–1854*, Philadelphia: University of Pennsylvania Press.

Bynum, William (1993) *Science and the Practice of Medicine in the Nineteenth Century*, Cambridge: Cambridge University Press.

Cain, P. J. and A. G. Hopkins (1993) *British Imperialism*, 2 vols, London: Longman.

Carter, K. Codell (1991) "The Development of Pasteur's Concept of Disease Causation and the Emergence of Specific Causes in 19th Century Medicine," *Bulletin of the History of Medicine and Allied Sciences* 65: 528–48.

Chandavarkar, Rajnarayan (1992) "Plague, Panic and Epidemic Politics in India, 1896–1914," in Terence Ranger and Paul Slack (eds) *Epidemics and Ideas: essays on the historical perception of pestilence*, Cambridge: Cambridge University Press.

Cunningham, Andrew (1992) "Transforming Plague. The laboratory and the identity of infectious disease," in Andrew Cunningham, Perry Williams (eds) *The Laboratory Revolution in Medicine*, Cambridge: Cambridge University Press.

Cunningham, Andrew and Perry Williams (1993) "De-centring the 'Big Picture': the origins of modern science and the modern origins of science," *British Journal for the History of Science* 12: 407–32.

Davis, Michael (2001) *Victorian Holocaust: El Nino*, New York: Verso.

Dormandy, Thomas (1999) *The White Death: a history of tuberculosis*, London: Hambledon Press.

Ernst, Waltraud and Bernard Harris (eds) (1999) *Race, Science and Medicine, 1700–1960*, London: Routledge.

Geison, Gerald (1995) *The Private Science of Louis Pasteur*, Princeton, NJ: Princeton University Press.

Hamlin, Christopher (1998) *Public Health and Social Justice in the Age of Chadwick, 1800–1854*, Cambridge: Cambridge University Press.

Have, Hank A. M. J. ten, G. K. Kimsma and S. F. Spicker (eds) (1990) *The Growth of Medical Knowledge*, Dordrecht: Kluwer Academic.

Hewlett, T. G. (1888) "Village Sanitation in India," India Office (London) V/23/69/337, Appendix G.

Huerkamp, Claudia (1990) "The Making of the Modern Medical Profession, 1800–1914: Prussian doctors in the nineteenth century," in Geoffrey Cocks and Konrad H. Jarausch (eds) *German Professions, 1800–1950*, New York: Oxford University Press.

Johnson, William (1995) *The Modern Epidemic: the history of TB in Japan*, Cambridge, MA: Harvard University Press.

Kearns, Gerry (1988) "Private Property and Public Health Reform in England 1830–70," *Social Science and Medicine* 26 (1): 187–99.

Kumar, Deepak (1997) "Unequal Contenders, Uneven Ground: medical encounters in British India, 1820–1920," in Andrew Cunningham (ed.) *Western Medicine as Contested Knowledge*, Manchester: Manchester University Press.

Lane, Joan (2001) *A Social History of Medicine: health, healing and disease in England, 1750–1950*, London: Routledge.

Lawrence, Christopher (1985) "Incommunicable Knowledge: science, technology and the clinical art in Britain 1850–1914," *Journal of Contemporary History* 20 (4): 503–20.

Lawrence, Christopher (2000) "Edward Jenner's Jockey Boots and the Great Tradition in English Medicine 1918–1939," in Christopher Lawrence and Anna-K. Mayer (eds) *Regenerating England: science, medicine and culture in inter-war Britain*, Amsterdam/Atlanta, GA: Rodopi.

Macleod, Roy M. (1967) "The Frustration of State Medicine, 1880–1899," *Medical History* 9: 19–31.

Muraleedharan, V. R. and D. Veeraraghaven (1992) "Anti-malarial policy in the Madras Presidency: an overview of the early decades of the twentieth century," *Medical History* 36: 290-305.

Porter, Dorothy and Roy Porter (1988) "The Politics of Prevention: anti-vaccinationism and public health in nineteenth century England," *Medical History* 32: 237–42.

Porter, Roy (1997) *The Greatest Benefit to Mankind*, London: HarperCollins.

Ramasubban, Radhika (1988) "Imperial Health in British India, 1857–1900," in Roy MacLeod and Milton Lewis (eds) *Disease, Medicine and Empire: perspectives on Western medicine and the experience of European expansion*, London: Routledge.

Rosner, Lisa (1991) *Medical Education in an Age of Improvement: Edinburgh students and apprentices 1760–1826*, Edinburgh: Edinburgh University Press.

Shapin, Stephen (1992) "Discipline and Bounding: the history and sociology of science as seen through the externalism-internalism debate," *History of Science* 30: 357–60.

Smith, F. B. (1979) *The People's Health 1830–1910*, New York: Holmes and Meier.

Stieglitz, Joseph (2002) *Globalization and its Discontents*, New York: W. W. Norton and Co.

Sturdy, Steve and Roger Cooter (1998) "Science, Scientific Management, and the Transformation of Medicine in Britain c. 1870–1950," *History of Science* 36: 421–66.

Szreter, Simon (1988) "The Importance of Social Intervention in Britain's Mortality Decline c. 1850–1914: a re-interpretation of the role of public health," *The Society for the Social History of Medicine* 1 (1–3): 1–37.

Trenn, T. J. and R. K. Merton (1979) (eds) *Ludwick Fleck: genesis and development of a scientific fact*, Chicago: University of Chicago Press.

Tuchman, Arleen (1993) *Science, Medicine and the State in Germany: the case of Baden 1815–1871*, Oxford: Oxford University Press.

Watts, Sheldon (1999) "British Development Policies and Malaria in India 1897–c.1929," *Past and Present* 165: 141–81.

Watts, Sheldon (2001) "From Rapid Changes to Stasis: official responses to cholera in British-ruled India and Egypt, 1800–1921," *Journal of World History* 12 (2): 321–74.

10 Health and medicine in the world, 1940 to the present

Alter, Joseph (1999) "Heaps of Health, Metaphysical Fitness: Ayurveda and the ontology of good health in medical anthropology," *Current Anthropology* 40 (supplement) S43–66. A post-colonial attack on biomedicine: with useful commentaries and bibliography.

Benedek, T. G. and J. Erlen (1999) "The Scientific Environment of the Tuskegee Study of Syphilis, 1920–1960," *Perspectives in Biology and Medicine* 43 (1): 1–30.

Cooter, Roger (ed.) (1988) *Studies in the History of Alternative Medicine*, Houndsmill, England: Macmillan.

Cunningham, Andrew and Perry Williams (eds) (1992) *The Laboratory Revolution in Medicine*, Cambridge: Cambridge University Press.

Davidson, Basil (1992) *The Black Man's Burden: Africa and the curse of the nation state*, New York: Times Books.

Falk, R. (1999) *Predatory Globalization*, Oxford: Polity.

Falola, Toyin and Dennis Ityavyar (1992) *The Political Economy of Health in Africa*, Athens, OH: University of Ohio Press.

Farmer, Paul (2001) *Infections and Inequalities: the modern plagues*, updated edition, Berkeley: University of California Press.

Feierman, Steven and John M. Janzen (eds) (1992) *The Social Basis of Health & Healing in Africa*, Berkeley: University of California Press.

Garrett, Laurie (1995) *The Coming Plague: newly emerging diseases in a world out of balance*, New York: Penguin.

Guerrant, Richard L. (1998) "Why America *must* care about Tropical Medicine: threats to global health and security from tropical infectious diseases," *American Journal of Tropical Medicine and Hygiene* 59 (1): 3–16.

Horton, Richard (2002) "Beyond the Cutting Edge," *Times Literary Supplement* 13 September 2002, 8–9.

Jütte, Robert (1999) "The Historiography of Nonconventional Medicine in Germany," *Medical History* 43: 342–58.

Leslie, Charles (1983) "New Research on Traditional Medicine in South Asia," *Social Science and Medicine* 17: 933–89.

Lurie, P., P. Hintzen and R. A. Lowe (1995) "Socioeconomic Obstacles to HIV Prevention and Treatment in Developing Countries: the roles of the International Monetary Fund and the World Bank," *AIDS* 9(6): 539–46.

McKeown, Edward (1976) *The Modern Rise of Population*, London: Edward Arnold.

O'Conner, Bonnie Blair (1995) *Healing Traditions: alternative medicine and the health profession*, University Park, PA: Pennsylvania University Press.

Park, Robert (2001) *Voodoo Science. The Road from Foolishness to Fraud*, New York: Oxford University Press.

Phillips, David R. and Yola Verhasselt (1994) "Health and Development: retrospect and prospects," in D. R. Phillips and Y. Verhasselt (eds) *Health and Development*, London: Routledge.

Porter, Roy (1997) *The Greatest Benefit to Mankind*, London: HarperCollins Publishers.

Porter, Roy (2002) *Madness: a brief history*, Oxford: Oxford University Press.

Ramsey, Matthew (1999) "Alternative Medicine in Modern France," *Medical History* 43: 286–322.

Shenk, David (2002) *The Forgetting: understanding Alzheimer's: a biography of a disease*, London: HarperCollins.

Sivin, Nathan (1987) *Traditional Medicine in Contemporary China*, Ann Arbor, MI: University of Michigan Press.

Sturdy, Steve and Roger Cooter (1998) "Science, Scientific Management and the Transformation of Medicine in Britain c. 1870–1950," *History of Science* 34: 421–66.

Tapper, Melbourne (1999) *In the Blood: sickle cell anemia and the politics of race*, Philadelphia: University of Pennsylvania Press.

Thomas, Patricia (2002) *Big Shot: passion, politics and the struggle for an AIDS vaccine*, Oxford: Public Affairs.

United Nations (annual) Development Reports using materials from the World Bank, the International Monetary Fund and other agencies.

Venkataramana, B. S. and P. V. Sarada (2001) "Extent and speed of spread of HIV infection in India through the commercial sex networks: a perspective," *Tropical Medicine & International Health* 6 (12): 1040–61.

Vitebsky, Piers (1993) "Is Death the Same Everywhere? Contexts of knowing and doubting," in Mark Hobart (ed.) *An Anthropological Critique of Development: the growth of ignorance*, London: Routledge.

Wellcome News (ed.) (2000) "Questioning the Alternative: complementary and alternative therapies," 23: Q2000.

Wilkinson, Richard (1996) *Unhealthy Societies, The Afflictions of Inequality*, London: Routledge.

World Health Organization (annual) *World Health Report*.

Index